On the Problem of Surrogate Parenthood

Analyzing the Baby M Case

On the Problem of Surrogate Parenthood

Analyzing the Baby M Case

---

edited by

HERBERT RICHARDSON

Symposium Series
Volume 25

The Edwin Mellen Press
Lewiston/Queenston

Library of Congress Cataloging-in-Publication Data

On the Problem of Surrogate Parenthood:
Analyzing the Baby M Case,
edited by Herbert Richardson

HQ
759.5
.O62
1987

This is volume 25 in the continuing series
Symposium Series
Volume 25 ISBN 0-88946-717-X
SS Series ISBN 0-88946-989-X

The Edwin Mellen Press   The Edwin Mellen Press
Box 450   Box 67
Lewiston, New York   Queenston, Ontario
USA 14092   L0S 1L0 CANADA

Printed in the United States of America

This book is dedicated to

Melissa Stern

LIST OF CONTRIBUTORS

Barbara Hilkert Andolsen
RUTGERS UNIVERSITY

H. E. Baber
UNIVERSITY OF SAN DIEGO

Henry M. Butzel
UNION COLLEGE

Mary Jo Deegan
UNIVERSITY OF NEBRASKA—LINCOLN

Marcus P. Ford
EUREKA COLLEGE

John Hamlin
UNIVERSITY OF MINNESOTA—DULUTH

Michael R. Hill
ALBION COLLEGE

Sandra B. Lubarsky
EUREKA COLLEGE

Jane Ollenburger
UNIVERSITY OF MINNESOTA—DULUTH

Herbert Richardson
UNIVERSITY OF TORONTO

Michael D. Ryan
DREW UNIVERSITY

Patricia H. Werhane
LOYOLA UNIVERSITY OF CHICAGO

N.B. The contributors for this volume are faculty at the above institutions which are listed for purposes of identification only. In accordance with the principles of academic freedom, the essays present the positions of the authors alone.

TABLE OF CONTENTS

A Guide to the Readings

The essays in this volume were written independently of one another in May, 1987, the month following Judge Sorkow's decision in the Baby "M" case. Because the trial itself, as well as its final outcome, divided members of the women's movement as well as legal and religious communities, it seemed a propitious moment when scholars might contribute to clarifying the issues. For this reason, I invited a number of experts in different fields to offer their reflections. Here is the result.

The two chief issues in the Baby "M" case were the legality of the surrogate contract and the custody of the child born from the surrogate relationship. Not surprisingly, therefore, the essays in this volume tend to focus on one or the other of these of two issues. A background problem, in several of the essays, is the legitimacy or desirability of the surrogate parenthood *per se*. Therefore, I have arranged the papers in this order of topics.

1) The first essay, by Professor Henry Butzel, provides a survey of the essential facts of the Baby "M" case and explains why Judge Sorkow had to deal with the two issues of the legitimacy of the contract and the custody decision together (though he had wanted to deal with them separately). Butzel explains:

> "Throughout the history of this case, the best intentions of the judge seem to have been thwarted. Initially he had hoped to bifurcate the issues and try the two parts of the case separately, first dealing with the legality of the surrogate contract. . . . [But] the higher court ruled that the issues could not be severed and the judge was thereby forced to consider both the legality of the contract and the custody issue simultaneously."

2) The second essay, by Professor Patricia Werhane, focuses on the issue of surrogate contracts and contends that they are *not* valid. Werhane's argument runs as follows:

"The idea of a contract is really questionable not only because (a) a mother cannot sell her baby (nor anyone else's for that matter), and because (b) a father (or anyone else) cannot buy it, but also because (c) in general, human beings have the very basic right not to be sold (or bought)."

3)   The third essay, by Professor Harriet Baber, presents arguments to support the validity of surrogacy contracts—the contrary view to that of the preceding essay. Baber says:

"Why should we not regard surrogate parent contracts as prenatal adoption papers? . . . Naturally, like agreements of any kind, surrogate parenting contracts may involve fraud or exploitation. This is, however, a good reason to make surrogate parenting contracts legally binding: by legalizing a practice we allow for the possibility of regulation and secure the protection of the law for all parties concerned."

4)   The fourth essay, by Professor Barbara Andolsen, moves beyond the discussion of the validity of the surrogate contract to a discussion of the historical and social changes shaping our modern notion of motherhood. She contends that "any acceptable policy to regulate surrogate contracts would have to include a provision guaranteeing a period of time after birth in which the surrogate could reconsider her decision to surrender the child."

Andolsen's argument about a "time for reconsideration" is based on her belief that the process of pregnancy itself is a necessary condition to making a valid decision. Hence, she contends that "no woman, even one who has borne a child before can give knowledgeable consent in advance to surrender her newborn." Further, Andolsen also notes that surrogacy tends to become a function of women who are at relative economic disadvantage; therefore, she points out the need for legal protection and social policies which will "insure that some (often economically vulnerable) women are not reduced to the status of merely useful uteri in order to gestate the children ardently desired by others."

5)   The fifth essay, by Professors Jane Ollenburger and John Hamlin, focuses specifically upon the issue of the economic exploitation of motherhood as a form of unpaid labor.

The authors point out that "women literally reproduce the labor force through childbirth." What the surrogacy contract does is to make explicit the fact that motherhood is a form of productive labor which should, as a matter of justice, be properly recompensed. "There has been enough volunteer motherhood."

Ollenburger and Hamlin are not sanguine about the possibilities of arranging just surrogate contracts.

"Class, gender and women of color divisions combine to create new forms of exploitation. Upper-middle and upper-class families can buy babies; lower-middle and, in some cases, lower class women can sell babies. However, socialist feminists should support surrogate mothering precisely because it does provide payment for labor that exists and until now has gone unpaid."

6) The sixth essay, by Professor Michael Hill, broadens the discussion immensely by introducing cross cultural considerations. Hill demonstrates that in all cultures, one must speak of multiple "forms of parenthood." He notes that every society distinguishes three forms of motherhood and three forms of fatherhood—the genetic, the gestational, and the educational—by presenting the following table:

Forms of Parenthood	
MALE	FEMALE
Genetic Father (contributes sperm)	Genetic Mother (contributes egg)
Genitor (provides supportive environment for pregnant genitrix)	Genitrix (provides gestation and/or supportive environment for pregnant genitrix)
Pater (provides care and socialization of child)	Mater (provides care and socialization of child)

On the basis of the above, Hill argues that Baby "M" has multiple parents and that "such multiple parent situations are not at all unusual. . . . Surrogate reproduction adds no new twists to parenting roles already in place and socially accepted."

7) The seventh essay, by Professor Mary Jo Deegan, presupposes the scheme of "multiple parenthood" outlined above. But Deegan argues that we do not have—and we desperately need—appropriate social rituals so that those who fulfill the surrogate mother role are properly acknowledged. Pointing out that a reason for the breakdown in the relation between the Whiteheads and the Sterns might have been the lack of an institutionalized ritual acknowledging the worth of the "gift mother" (surrogate mother), Deegan then attempts to construct this kind of ritual which would help sustain—on psychological, social, and religious levels—the practice of surrogacy:

"In 1906, Arnold Van Gennepp (1966) articulated for Western society the rich and varied world of rituals in nonmodern societies. His work has been elaborated by Victor Turner in a series of books (e.g., 1967, 1969, 1974, 1982). Both theorists examine rites of passage as processual, with ceremonies of *separation, maginality* (or *liminality*), and *reaggregation.* Turner and Van Gennepp's ideas organize my ideas for surrogate mothering as a celebration of a birth and its gift of love from one family to another."

8) The eighth essay, by Professor Michael Ryan, introduces the idea of "religious" (as distinct from "secular") motivations for surrogate motherhood. Noting that the basic motivation of Mrs. Whitehead was "to give an infertile mother the gift of a child so that God might perhaps give a child to an infertile relative of hers [i.e., Mrs. Whitehead's]," Ryan contrasts this religious motivation with the motivation of a woman "renting out her body . . . merely for money." The problem, Ryan notes, is that a person can be motivated *both* ways because our motivations are not simple and it is quite possible that people may not be fully clear about their intentions—and may even change or reformulate them in the course of pregnancy. This means, for Ryan, that the key issue is the *sorting out* motivations so as to arrive at a sense of personal integrity we can live with.

9) The ninth essay, by Professor Herbert Richardson, argues that the dominant tendency of our society is to interpret procreation as an activity whereby parents "produce" children as if they were things. Richardson argues that the Catholic (and religious) interpretation of children as a "gift from God" is the best protection against regarding children as "things" whose rights derive from society. Though Richardson argues in behalf of the Catholic creationist position, he does not follow that Church's admonition against "interference" with natural procreative processes. Instead, he argues that medical technology (and *in vitro* fertilization) can provide a no less "moral" condition in relation to which God can create "souls" as the act of natural intercourse. He says:

> "If the qualifying condition for conception is human activity which creates and expresses love, then this love need not be identified only with the act of sexual intercourse. Rather, this love may be expressed through a variety of other means such as *in vitro* fertilization. . . . There is no reason at all why God may not be conceived to act in relation to such scientific activity if God may also be conceived to act in relation to nature and to natural activity."

10) The tenth essay, by Professors Marcus Ford and Sandra Lubarsky, offers a critique of various notions of the family. They argue that, in that last analysis, what is most important is the "organic family, that is, the web of human relationships which include bonds with persons with whom one shares no "blood." From this perspective, the authors regard surrogacy as a practice presupposing notions ("genetic identity," "blood brotherhood") which fall beneath the universalistic orientation toward all humanity to which we should aspire. "Surrogate motherhood (or, more accurately, prearranged adoption of a genetically-related child) undercuts what we understand to be the most fundamental sense of the family, the organic meaning, by giving undue credence to the biological and the legal notions of the family." Therefore, Ford and Lubarsky argue that surrogacy is an undesirable practice at this time.

—Editor

The Essential Facts
of the BABY M Case

HENRY M. BUTZEL

I. Introduction

"Now Sarai, Abram's wife, bore him no children. She had an Egyptian maid whose name was Hagar; and Sarai said to Abram, 'Behold now, the Lord has prevented me from bearing children; go in to my maid; it may be that I shall obtain children by her'" (Genesis 16). The case referred to there also had unfortunate results initially. "And Sarai said to Abram, 'may the wrong done to me be on you! I gave my maid to your embrace, and when she saw that she had conceived, she looked on me with contempt.'...And the angel of the Lord said to her [Hagar], 'Behold you are with child, and shall bear a son; you shall call his name Ishmael...He shall be a wild ass of a man, his hand against every man and every man's hand against him...'." Later, of course the story has a less unfortunate outcome as Abram (now Abraham) and Sarai (now Sarah), despite their being in their 90's, bear their own children. And, of course, America's most famous novel will begin, "Call me Ishmael." One can see that the practice of surrogate motherhood certainly is not new.

Ordinarily one would prefer not to comment upon a legal suit which is still under adjudication, as it might be construed as an attempt to interfere with justice, or an attempt to intercede where one has no legal standing. However, in this particular case, due in part to the actions of one of the parties concerned, there has been sufficient intervention and comment by the press so as to spread the day-to-day record, as well as part of the trial judge's opinion at the conclusion of the case, before the public and the usual restraints seem invalid. Nonetheless, these remarks will limit themselves, when discussing the actual case, to those statements presented in the judge's opinion, and will not base any material, factual or conjectural, upon the more than 100 press clippings in my collection of remarks about this case.

Perhaps it is also not necessary to present a cast of characters after all of this publicity. But for the sake of clarity let us remember we deal with 5 principle characters, Baby "M", the central figure in this case, Mr. and Mrs. Whitehead, the surrogate mother and her husband, and Mr. and Mrs. Stern, the would-be legal parents of the infant. In reality, in the legal aspects of this case only Mrs. Whitehead, the surrogate and biological mother, and Mr. Stern, the sperm donor and biological father, of the child play a role. In addition other characters include the two Whitehead children born several years ago, and Catherine and Joseph Messer, the parents of Mrs. Whitehead. And of course, the judge, Harvey R. Sorkow, plays a major role in the case.

The events of this case leading up to the trial are somewhat complex, and perhaps the following chronology will help orient the reader in following the logic of the events leading up to the judge's decision.

DATE	EVENT
6/2/73	Whiteheads married; she 16, he 24. Two children, a son in 1974, and a daughter in 1976.
6/27/74	Sterns married; both are 28 years old.
1976	Mr. Whitehead has a vasectomy as the couple are satisfied that a family of two, one boy and one girl, is "ideal."
1978	Whiteheads separate briefly.
1983	Whiteheads declare bankruptcy.
4/84	Mrs. Whitehead receives psychological screening for the surrogacy program.
5/84	Mrs. Whitehead matched with a couple, *not* the Sterns.
5/84	Mrs. Whitehead sees her lawyer and signs a surrogate contract, with slight changes from standard form supplied by the Infertility Clinic of New York (ICNY), with the above couple.
8/84	Sterns look for surrogacy.
12/84	Sterns sign up with ICNY.
1/85	Whiteheads meet the Sterns.
2/85	Mrs. Whitehead signs contract with Mr. Sterns. She does not consult her lawyer; Mrs. Stern and Mr. Whitehead not signatories.

7/85	After nine attempts fertilization occurs.
3/27/86	Baby M born. Mr. Whitehead's name goes on birth certificate. First name of child on birth certificate is furnished by Mrs. Whitehead, and is not the name selected by Sterns for child, a two-fold violation of contract.
3/27/86	Mr. Stern visits hospital; not allowed to hold child as he is not listed as father on birth certificate.
3/28/86	First indication of trouble; Mrs. Whitehead not sure she can give up child.
3/30/86	Mrs. Whitehead takes child home.
3/30/86	Sterns come to Whiteheads' home and recover child.
3/31/86	Mrs. Whitehead comes to Sterns and asks to have baby for one week. The Sterns agree as Mrs. Whitehead seems so distraught they are apparently concerned for her mental health.
4/1/86	Mrs. Whitehead informs Sterns she will be away and unavailable for a week. Actually she takes baby out of state to visit her parents in Florida. Her parents up to this time do not know she is genetic mother, but think that she carried an *in vitro* embryo.
4/8/86	Mrs. Whitehead returns to New Jersey. Promises to return child on 4/12.
4/11/86	Mrs. Whitehead informs Sterns she wants more time.
4/12/86	Sterns visit; Mrs. Whitehead informs them she intends to keep child.
4/20/86	Whiteheads' house up for sale; apparently they are planning to move to Florida.
5/5/86	Court order for return of baby to Sterns.
5/5/86	In mixup while attempting to serve writ and obtain baby, police accidentally allow baby to be passed out the back window to Mr. Whitehead and baby is now gone.
5/6/86	Whiteheads to Florida for 87 days first staying at her parents. During this time no post-natal vaccination or other normal medical procedures are undertaken by Mrs. Whitehead.

5/20/86	Whiteheads in 15 different motels in 20 days to avoid police. Their daughter is enrolled in Florida schools.
7/15/86	Call to Sterns from Mrs. Whitehead. She threatens suicide and murder of child.
7/21/86	Mrs. Whitehead's mother calls in press.
7/28/86	Mrs. Whitehead enters hospital for unlisted cause; Mr. Whitehead returns child to grandparents.
7/31/86	Florida police take custody of baby.
8/1/86	Mrs. Whitehead holds press conference in hospital.
8/6-16/86	First lawyers for Whiteheads hired.
8/13/86	Court appoints *guardian ad litem* for baby.
9/2/86	Mrs. Whitehead attempts to bring counterclaim and accuses Sterns of fraud.
10/7/86	Grandparents enter case demanding visitation rights.
10/20/86	Mrs. Whitehead's visitations allowed to be increased.
11/18/86	Trial set for 1/5/87.
12/3/86	Superior court refuses to allow judge to bifurcate issues in trial.

Further dicussion now seems naturally to divide itself into three parts; first the *genetic* issues will be discussed, then some of the *legal* issues and past precedents for them will presented. Finally a few remarks upon the entire subject of surrogacy will be offered.

II. Genetic Issues

There should be no apparent genetic issues involved in this case; surrogate motherhood of this type is the same in terms of genetic results as Artificial Insemination, Donor (AID). The offspring born in either manner receive 1/2 of her or his genes from the mother and 1/2 from the father. The legal and genetic issues surrounding AID have long been resolved; such children are considered fully legitimate under the law; that is the husband is legally responsible for the child (People vs. Sorensen, u437 P. 2d 495, 1968). This type of genetic issue should therefore not have played any part in the Baby M case. However, initially a genetic role seemed possible as the surrogate mother, Mrs. Whitehead, claimed to have had intercourse with her husband without the use of contraceptive devices at about the same time as the artificial insemination with Mr. Stern's sperm was performed. The court ordered an HLA antigen test for determination of paternity, legal in the state of New Jersey, (Malvasi v. Malvasi, 401 A.2d 279, 1979) and it was found the probability of the surrogate's husband being the father of the infant was zero, and that Mr. Stern showed a probability of **98% of being the father. (The claim by Mrs. Whitehead for paternity by her spouse was later to shown to be in itself improbable as Mr. Whitehead had undergone a vasectomy some years previously! See chronicle of events above.)

In this case both Mrs. Whitehead and Mr. Stern therefore correctly share a genetic relationship to the infant.

Additionally, it will be contested whether Mrs. Stern is truly incapable of child-bearing, or even that she may have some genetic defect which she does not wish to pass on to her offspring. Also it might be noted that Mrs. Stern is at the age where an offspring's risk of chromosomal disease, such as Down syndrome, is significantly higher than it would be were the mother at a younger age.

Be that as it may, there can be other genetic problems in surrogate motherhood. For example, it is today possible to carry out *in vitro* fertilizations and to obtain and store viable embryos for longer periods of time. At the appropriate time such embryos, which may have no genetic relationship to either the surrogate mother or the family desiring a child, may be implanted in the womb of a surrogate mother for normal gestation. Here the use of a surrogate might be due to the woman who produced the egg being unable to carry a child because of physiological or morphological defects. It is even possible that the couple using a surrogate might have no genetic relationship to the stored embryo. The resulting offspring now has no genetic relationship with any of the persons involved in its gestation. Should a dispute arise as to custody of this infant, neither side can make use of genetic claims of parenthood.

Further, at least one case is known in which the offspring of a surrogate "union" was *not* genetically related to the supposed sperm donor. In this instance, unfortunately, the resultant child was born with multiple severe birth defects, essentially being born without a brain. Blood tests were ordered, resulting in the elimination of the sperm donor as a possible father. The question arose as to who was legally and financially responsible for the child now that it had been born. Obviously, the sperm donor did not want this child, the so-called surrogate mother did not want the child, nor was the child of a type who could be readily placed into adoption. However, had the blood tests shown that the sperm donor was genetically the father of the child then he might have been held responsible under a surrogate contract for the costs of rearing the child until its early demise.

Still another possible scenario could be imagined in which the sperm used to inseminate the surrogate mother could have come from a sperm bank and from a sperm donor who is not the man signing the surrogate contract. In this case, the surrogate mother would have a genetic relationship to the child, but the man who signed the contract would not.

Thus, genetics does play a role in decisions involving surrogacy. There are, as pointed out, several possible results; 1) both the surrogate mother and the sperm donor contribute equally to the genetic makeup of the resulting child; 2) neither the surrogate nor the sperm donor contribute any genetic material to the child, or; 3) the surrogate mother will contribute genetic material but the man signing the contract will not contribute genetic material. It would seem that in any dispute over the resulting offspring the genetic contribution would play some role in the decision-making process.

III. Legal Aspects

"SURROGATE MOTHER WANTED. Couple unable to have child willing to pay $10,000.00 fee and expenses to woman to carry husband's child. Conception by artificial insemination. All replies confidential."

It was the above advertisement by the ICNY in the *Asbury Park Press* to which Mrs. Whitehead replied, thereby setting this case in motion. Mrs. Whitehead then received a brochure defining female infertility and listing "medical reasons" as one of the conditions for a woman seeking a surrogate mother.

Before examining the opinion in this case, it should be pointed out that there have been previous court cases involving surrogate motherhood. Decisions in other states, one in Michigan (*Doe v. Kelley*, 307 N.W.2d 438, 1981) and one in Kentucky (*Surrogate Parenting Association Inc. vs. Commonwealth of Kentucky*, Supreme Court slip opinion, 85-SC-421-DG, 1986). These, of course, lack validity as precedents in New Jersey, but are of interest because of the fact that they are directly opposite. The first case, decided by the Supreme Court of Michigan in 1981 ruled that surrogate contracts were illegal and violated the adoption laws of that state. The second case, in 1986 was decided by the Supreme Court of Kentucky, and ruled the contracts were legally valid, as adoption played no role in such a contract. As the child's biological father is the one signing the contract, his wife is not a party to the contract. There is no need, nor can there be, for an adoption by him; the father cannot adopt his own child. The adoption laws therefore may not apply to surrogacy. What happens after the father takes his child, usually an adoption by the mother, is *not* part of the contract; indeed the woman does not sign the document; only the father and the surrogate mother are parties to the contract. While unlikely, it should be pointed out that as far as the contract is concerned, the father need not even be married!

Unfortunately for all in this case, but mostly for Baby "M," the single, most important legal issue, namely custody of the infant, decided by a judge on the basis of what is *the best interest of the child*, became hopelessly entangled with other legal issues, all of which should be secondary in making that primary decision. The issue whether the surrogate contract is voided by the Adoption Laws which specifically prohibit the payment of any money for adoption, as well as also forbidding the signing away of parental rights until 5 days after the birth of a child, is a valid issue, but still not the major one. For, as the judge pointed out, the importance of the *parens patria* decision was utmost; the judge could award custody of the child to either the Sterns or the Whiteheads regardless of the legality of the contract.

There were also attempts to prove fraud on the part of Mrs. Stern, listed in the contract as being unable to bear a child. In *sensu strictu* she was not incapable of bearing a child, but she did not wish to risk a pregnancy as she has a mild case of multiple sclerosis. Medical experts who testified during the trial suggested that a pregnancy might exacerbate this illness to a serious degree, possibly seriously endangering Mrs. Stern's health.

Also, as already mentioned, an attempt was made to disprove the paternity of Mr. Stern and to fall back upon the formerly almost iron-clad rule that a child born to a married couple was presumed to be legitimate regardless of the biological paternity of the husband or of another man. Only with the introduction of the Human Leucocyte Antigen (HLA) tests could this be legally disputed, and it is of interest to note that New Jersey was among the first states to take judicial notice of this method.

Throughout the history of this case, the best intentions of the judge seem to have been thwarted. Initially he had hoped to bifurcate the issues and try the two parts of the case separately, first dealing with the legality of the surrogate contract. Should he find it legal, and his decision upheld by the superior courts, then there might be no further need for other legal procedures dealing with custody as the contract specified that Mr. Stern would receive custody of the child.

Should the contract be held void, he would then deal with the case as a normal custody trial dealing with an illegitimate child, deciding custody on the basis of what would be the best interest of the child. This would normally take place in a closed court with only the participants present, here the Sterns and the Whiteheads, and the *guardian ad litem* for the infant. A decision would be reached by the judge and the entire proceedings would be *in camera* to protect the best interests of the child in the future.

Unfortunately both intentions were frustrated. The higher court ruled that the issues could not be severed and the judge was thereby forced to consider both the legality of the contract and the custody issue simultaneously. Second, the issue of a closed trial became moot as first the grandparents of the child, and then the surrogate mother herself, held extensive press conferences concerning the case. Both conferences were held in Florida, the first upon the return of Baby M to the grandparents after the Whiteheads had stayed at various motels in Florida for several weeks in order to avoid the legally mandated return of the child to the Sterns. Probably the only reason for the baby's return was the fact that for reasons not given in the opinion, Mrs. Whitehead entered a Florida hospital. It was while she was in the hospital that the 2nd press conference was held at her request. Although both the press interviews were held in Florida, the New York and New Jersey papers picked the story up quickly and it "exploded" into a barrage of further articles, interviews, etc. (I have over 140 various newspaper and magazines articles or stories covering this case, and this does not count the extensive television coverage given it.) There could no longer be any reason to close the custody hearings as the facts were already so widely disseminated that no real benefit to the child would be served by a closed hearing.

The trial itself lasted six weeks and the judge's opinion of 121 pages dealt with many different facets of the case. Among these was the judge's evaluation of the 38 expert and lay witnesses testifying for one or the other party or for the *guardian ad litem*. Judge Sorkow found that some witnesses offered by the Whiteheads simply were not credible; i.e., the credentials presented by one did not seem to qualify her to render an opinion in the case. Another witness was found by the judge to be misinterpreting her role, as "Her testimony centers on the adult while the only concern of the court is the child."

A third witness's testimony was "totally discounted" as it was found that she had written a letter to the court, signing Mrs. Whitehead's name and " ...a transcript of her apparently perjurious testimony was referred to the Bergen County Prosecutor." Still other "experts" presented by Mrs. Whitehead seemed less than credible in the eyes of Judge Sorkow.

Among the duties of a judge in a custody case is to investigate the background of the two contestants seeking the child. Here there is a vast difference between the two families. The judge went to considerable lengths, in deciding to grant custody to the Sterns, to point out these differences, noting the educational background of the couples involved. Both the Sterns had PhD's, and Mrs. Stern in addition was an M.D. Mrs. Whitehead did not finish high school, and at one time had removed her son from school when she disagreed with the manner in which he was being treated. The court also inquired into the emotional stability, financial stability, regard for education as well as the attitudes of the various parties towards the child as a person or as an extension of their own personality.

In fact, in almost every regard, two more disparate couples would be hard to find. Both the Sterns testified as to how they planned the upbringing of the child and how they had reorganized their lives so as to make certain the child would "grow up as a private person in a loving home." The judge found that Mrs. Whitehead did not offer the same caring provisions for raising the child as an individual. Surprisingly, although he was readily available throughout the trial, Mr. Whitehead was never called to testify. Given all the evidence before him, it is not difficult to see why Judge Sorkow would award custody to the Sterns.

In addition, the legality of the surrogate contract was established by the judge, on a basis similar to that used by the Kentucky Supreme Court mentioned previously. The judge examined the terms of the contract carefully, and noted that there was no coercion involved and that up to the time Mrs. Whitehead conceived she could have voluntarily removed herself from the terms of the contract. Once conception occurred, however, then she was bound to fulfill the contract and to give the resultant child to Mr. Stern. The judge, however, did rule one section of the contract illegal, namely the clause prohibiting abortion of the fetus without Mr. Stern's permission. He noted that this was contrary to the U.S. Supreme Court abortion decision giving a woman absolute control of her body and the clause in the contract dealing with this matter was unconstitutional. As this did not in any way enter into the suit, this change was of no consequence in the decision. The agreement giving Mr. Stern the right to have his name listed as the father of the child and to select a name for the child and to be given custody of the child after her birth was held to be a valid contract. Thus with both the custody and the contract issue the Sterns emerged as the winners of the case. It seems worthwhile here to quote the last paragraphs of Judge Sorkow's opinion: "It was said Melissa needs an end to litigation, she needs to have her parentage fixed, she needs protection from anyone who would threaten her protection, so as not to be manipulated and she needs a strong support system to protect her privacy.

"It was also said it is not in Melissa's best interest to have such public attention and scrutiny of her life. Common sense and common decency require that what Melissa must learn, she must learn in a very private manner.

"Melissa needs stability and peace, so that she can be nurtured in a loving environment free from chaos and sheltered from the public eye.

"This court says that Melissa deserved nothing less -- stability and peace" (Superior Court of New Jersey, Chancery Division/Family Part Bergen County, Docket No. FM-25314-86E).

Judge Sorkow went one step further, however. After his decision he called the Sterns into his chambers and carried out an adoption procedure whereby the original birth certificate, listing the wrong father and the wrong name for the child, was invalidated and a new certificate listing Mr. Stern as the father and the Sterns' name for the child, Melissa, was filed. In addition, with the granting of the adoption by Mrs. Stern, all parental and grand-parental visitation rights for Mrs. Whitehead and her parents were legally terminated.

Unfortunately for Melissa, cases such as these never seem to end quickly. The case is presently under appeal and the court dockets are so loaded that even with the most expeditious handling of the case, it will not be until September, 1987 that the appeal will come before the superior court. (By the time the final appeals are decided, Melissa will be almost 2 years old.) Meanwhile, the appellate court court has restored visitation rights to Mrs. Whitehead pending the final outcome of the appeal. In addition, further complications are arising; Mrs. Whitehead's parents are again requesting visitation rights also, and Mrs. Whitehead is claiming that Judge Sorkow should have been disqualified as he is "biased." One cannot predict the final outcome of this case; one can only be certain that the concern for privacy and a quiet life for Melissa is not soon to come.

III. General Remarks

It would seem that in one form or another, the practice of surrogate motherhood is likely to continue. There are some features which should be pointed out, some of them so strongly evident in this case. Others, while perhaps not a direct factor in the Baby M decision also must be considered. Indeed even the Michigan Court which deemed surrogate contracts to be invalid pointed out that surrogate motherhood without payment to the mother is not an illegal practice and does not come under jurisdiction of the courts. Obviously in these cases, no contract is necessary, or, should there be one, it would specify that no payment other than medical and hospital costs will be made.

Assuming that payment for surrogate mothers becomes generally legally acceptable, what further precautions need be taken? It should be noted that this is not the first instance of a surrogate mother deciding to keep a child after it has been born. Noel Keane, a lawyer and the foremost advocate of the practice of surrogate motherhood, refers in his book to a woman who fled to California with her child, and at the time he wrote the book there had been no recovery by the biological father whose name was on the birth certificate for the infant. (Keane, N.P. with Breo, D. L. 1981. The Surrogate Mother, Everest House, New York.)

There indeed seems to be a genuine problem in the selection of the proper women as surrogate mothers. Indeed, in this case there is evidence that the psychological screening of Mrs. Whitehead showed some doubt whether she would be able to give up a child after its birth; unfortunately this was not followed up. But, given the 9 months' pregnancy and the drama of birth, there may be a real biological question whether bonding of mother to child makes the act of surrendering the infant to another couple unnatural. Particularly in this case, where Mrs. Whitehead did not inform the hospital of the true circumstances of the child's conception, thereby having her husband's name entered upon the birth certificate and being able to take the child home from the hospital, such a bonding may seem possible.

Particularly in the case of a surrogate mother with possible emotional problems, bonding, imaginary or real, might be more likely to occur. In addition then to the present screening practice for selection of these women, including past fertility and apparent willingness to accept both the responsibility of a pregnancy and the monetary rewards thereof, a much more in-depth psychological history probably should be an essential for acceptance into the program. Perhaps, had this been done the case of Baby M might never have arisen. There are many former surrogate mothers who have given up their children, some of whom presently may have regrets, but none of whom have gone to court. This might imply that the previous and present screening program of would-be surrogate mothers is adequate; however this case indicates that screening must be done more carefully. Even the slightest doubt concerning the willingness of the birth mother to surrender the child upon birth, possibly without even seeing the infant, should automatically disqualify the surrogate.

It would seem that in many instances a woman offering to be a surrogate mother is genuinely interested in helping infertile couples. In such cases, the monetary incentive may not be necessary. Indeed, the payments beyond medical and hospital expenses may be offered only in order to expand the availability of such women and thereby allow the practice of surrogate motherhood to continue and to grow.

This then raises an issue which might be much more important than it has been in the past, namely who should be in charge of arranging surrogate contracts and what should the reward for this service be? It is obvious that clinics and legal services are costly, but wht should be the ratio between the amount paid to the surrogate mother and to the clinic be? In the first instance, a woman has agreed to a 9-months contract, 24 hours a day, and with several restrictions upon what she can or cannot do during the pregnancy. On the other hand the clinic and its legal arm have expended probably not much more than the equivalent of a few days' time; to what extent should they be reimbursed compared to amount paid the surrogate mother? Granted neither the would-be parents nor the surrogate mother would be likely to find each other without the existence of the clinic, but should the latter be a public service with costs reimbursed by the users or the state, or should the clinic be allowed to be run as a for-profit organization?

Still another problem seems to emerge with this case. Obviously Mrs. Whitehead has had considerable legal counsel, three lawyers during a long trial. Yet she is in no position to offer them the amount of money which their time would seem to demand. Even were she to win the case, there are no monetary damages to be awarded from which counsel can be paid. The great disparity between the income of the couple desiring the child and the surrogate mother in this, and probably other cases, almost insures which side will be able to afford the more costly legal fees. Unless the surrogate mother can in some way use the proceedings of the legal case to assure her of income, such as movie, television, or book rights, her lawyers may indeed go unpaid.

Yet the need for her to raise money in one or more of these manners patently defeats the very purpose expressed so clearly by Judge Sorkow at the end of his opinion, namely the privacy of the child.

One result of this case may be salutory; many states are at the moment considering legislation which would deal with surrogate motherhood. New York, for example, has seen the preparation of three different bills, ranging from absolute prohibition to granting of legality to cases exactly like this one, but with the consent of a court. Probably no action will be taken here as it is near the end of the legislative session, and other matters have higher priority in the time remaining before adjournment. Nonetheless the Baby M case has brought the issue to the fore, and perhaps some statutory guidelines in various states will help to avoid this type of case in the future. Certainly for any child born as result of *legalized* surrogate motherhood there will be the privacy and "stability and peace" sought by Judge Sorkow. This case, then, while it almost certainly cannot but harm Melissa for some time, may in the long run provide several useful precedents for the future. For one thing it will certainly provoke lengthy and sometimes acerbic discussions over not only the legality of surrogate motherhood, but also over the moral and religious issues involved. The decision by Judge Sorkow will be a landmark in cases such as this, and the readers of this discussion are strongly urged to study it with care. It sets forth all of the issues, perhaps sets a model for future decisions, and certainly shows an attempt to end the case in a humane manner solely for the future benefit of Melissa. One cannot, as said earlier, predict what the higher courts will do, but regardless of their decision, Judge Sorkow's opinion will provide either a model for future cases, or a model for dissenting opinions should such cases arise. Often dissenting opinions some years later become majority opinions in new trials; perhaps in the future Judge Sorkow's thoughtful opinion in this case will eventually become the authoritative source upon which all other cases are firmly based.

AGAINST the Legitimacy
of Surrogate Contracts

PATRICIA H. WERHANE

Come away, O Human child!
To the waters and the wild
With a faery, hand in hand,
For the world's more full of weeping
than you can understand.[1]

One initial reaction to the issue of surrogate motherhood as it presents itself in the Baby M case is that such arrangements between unmarried natural parents are at best strange, and at worst unnatural. But such an intuitive feeling will not serve as an argument against such arrangements not only because it is not an *argument*, but also because, ever since humankind discovered fire, and perhaps even earlier, we have been interfering with nature by performing and perpetuating strange and even unnatural acts. So I shall spend some time mustering arguments against the practice of this form of surrogate motherhood. These arguments may not be conclusive as applied to the Baby M case, but if they make sense, these conclusions have serious implications for other similar situations.

I want to distinguish surrogate motherhood in the Baby M case from other practices of *in vitro* fertilization and artificial insemination. One may use the term "genetic motherhood" and "genetic fatherhood" to refer to the contribution (or sale) of one's ova or sperm. The term "gestational motherhood" will refer to the activity of carrying a fetus including the implantation of a fertilized egg into the womb of a third party. It is obvious that one can be a genetic "parent" without being a gestational mother and vice versa. I shall not discuss the moral implications of mere genetic or gestational "parenthood" nor whether or not individually one of these constitutes full parenthood. Natural motherhood, as I shall use the term, constitutes genetic and gestational motherhood wherein one carries one's own fertilized ovum. Similarly, natural fatherhood constitutes the deliberate implantation of one's sperm into a chosen natural mother. One should also distinguish nurturing mothers and nurturing fathers, those person or persons who raise the child. Finally, surrogate motherhood, at least in theory, should constitute being a substitute mother, in any one of the ways just enumerated.

The case of Baby M and cases like it involve artificial insemination of the sperm of the natural father into the natural mother who is also the surrogate for the nurturing mother, because the natural mother promises to give up the baby at birth to the prospective nurturing mother and the natural father. So Mrs. Whitehead, the natural mother of Baby M, is both a natural and a surrogate mother. In the Baby M case the arrangement involved a written contract between the natural mother, the natural father, and the natural father's wife, but there probably are countless other instances where there was merely an agreement without a contract. In this case too, the conception entailed artificial insemination, but traditionally such motherhood might entail a sexual relationship between the natural parents.

The Baby M case raises a number of issues. First, what is the binding nature and extent of a contract (written or unwritten) made between consenting adults, in this case a contract whereby Baby M would be given up to the Sterns at birth? When or can such contracts override individual rights, societal good, or other interests? Secondly, does the fact of natural motherhood extend special rights to the natural mother? Are her claims equal to, less than, or greater than, those of the natural father? Or can either or both parental claims to Baby M be set aside when certain agreements are made? Third, what are the rights of the baby in this situation? Do any of these rights claims override a contract freely agreed upon by rational consenting adults? Finally, can surrogate motherhood be justified on utilitarian or other grounds?

Let us begin by focusing on the contract made between Mrs. Whitehead and the Sterns. In the early twentieth century, from 1905 until 1937, the notion of "freedom of contract" had almost an absolute binding force in the law and in the courts. The principle, firmly established by a famous Supreme Court case, *Lockner v. New York* in 1905, ruled that the due processes clauses of the Constitution (principally the Fifth and Fourteenth Amendments) protect freedom of contract and therefore protect the freedom of people to make binding agreements of their choice.[2] A contract entered into voluntarily by two or more consenting rational adults is a binding one, not to be overridden by other considerations nor by the courts or other laws.

> . . . [F]reedom of contract is . . . the general rule and restraint the exception; and the exercise of legislative authority to abridge it can be justified only by the existence of exceptional circumstances.[3]

The Lockner case is cited specifically by the Baby M court as protecting the rights of both parties, Mrs. Whitehead and Mr. Stern, voluntarily to enter into the surrogate motherhood contract. It is also cited as a precedent for holding this contract as a binding one.[4] Yet *Lockner* specifically dealt with striking down labor laws because they allegedly interfere with "the general right of an individual to be free in his person and his power to contract in relation to his own labor."[5] This means that Lockner protects the freedom of employees and employers to make work agreements of their choice. But the Baby M court surely cannot mean that because Baby M is a result of Mrs. Whitehead's labor, she has the right to do with Baby M as she pleases including the right to enter into an agreement to sell her. So the New Jersey Court must be appealing to *Lockner* on other grounds.

While the Lockner decision establishes and protects freedom of contract in a wide area, subsequent decisions based on the Lockner decision make it clear that "[t]here is . . . no such thing as absolute freedom of contract"[6] specifically when one is dealing with human health and well-being. Moreover, the scope of application of freedom of contract as interpreted by the Lockner court was challenged in another famous Supreme Court case, *West Coast Hotel v. Parrish*,[7] in 1937, and since that 1937 decision the alleged binding nature of freedom of contract has been under constant attack by legal experts and overruled countless times in the courts.[8]

Admittedly, the Baby M contract was freely drawn up by both parties with full knowledge of its consequences. Yet the early Constitutional prohibition against voluntary slavery and indenture, the fact that *Lockner* specifically deals with freedom of contract in labor agreements, and the subsequent string of decisions after *Lockner* that narrowed the scope of freedom of contract undermine the appeal to *Lockner* as a good defense of the Baby M contract. Should a contract, *any* contract, be legally or morally binding even when it is entered into voluntarily by both parties when and if it entails selling, renting, or indenturing a human being? Despite the New Jersey Court's defense of the legality and binding nature of the contract between Mrs. Whitehead and the Sterns, one's intuitive reaction is that it should not, and there is a great deal of legal and moral precedent to support that intuition.

The court in the Baby M case argued further that the Constitution protects the right to privacy including the right to procreate. According to the court, under the substantive due process clauses of the Fourteenth Amendment this includes equal protection of *means* of reproduction including the right to enter into "reproductive contracts" since

refusal to enforce these contracts and prohibition of money payments would constitute an unconstitutional interference with procreative liberty since it would prevent childless couples from obtaining the means with which to have families.[9]

This interpretation allows equal protection for a variety of means of reproduction including ova or sperm donors, *in vitro* fertilization, artificial insemination, use of third-party wombs and other advanced techniques to aid in reproduction. The New Jersey court argued further that

protected means extends to the use of surrogates. The contract cannot fall because of the use of a third party . . . [R]efusal to enforce these [surrogate motherhood] contracts and prohibition of money payments would constitute an unconstitutional interference with procreative liberty since it would prevent childless couples from obtaining the means with which to have families.[10]

Because sperm donation or sale is legal, so, too, a woman must equally be able to offer for sale a "means for procreation."[11] That is what Mrs. Whitehead did, so that contract must be protected just as a contract of a sperm donor is protected under the law.

Reproductive contracts which entail artificial insemination or *in vitro* fertilization, that is, the liberty to experiment with various *means* of reproduction, can be defended or criticized depending on who is involved and the circumstances under which the activity takes place. One cannot defend or criticize the Baby M case on the basis of artificial insemination. Selling of donating ova or sperm, or "renting a womb," might be justified on the grounds that mere genetic motherhood or fatherhood or mere gestational motherhood does not constitute full parenthood. In the former, one is not choosing the genetic partner; in the latter, one is not genetically involved. So genetic and gestational parents might not have full rights to their offspring for these reasons. On these grounds, one might be able to justify Mrs. Whitehead's surrogacy if she had merely donated ova *or* been a gestational mother.

The Baby M case, however, is different. Mrs. Whitehead is the genetic, the gestational, and thus the natural mother of Baby M. Whether or not parenthood or full parenthood could be granted to a genetic parent or to a gestational parent, I would defend the view that the combination, at least, constitutes full parenthood. Mrs. Whitehead and Mr. Stern have full rights as natural parents of Baby M. But if one interprets the liberty to procreate as the right of natural parents to make binding contracts which cannot be overturned including contracts to buy or sell their natural child, then the Baby M decision places the rights to be adoptive parents as preempting the rights of the natural mother, the natural father, or for that matter, the rights of the child. According to this line of reasoning, it is justified to buy or sell a child, even your own natural child, if this arrangement is a contractual one, if it satisfies your desires or the desires of other people to be parents? Any contract to do so forfeits your parental rights. This implies that equal protection of surrogate parenting under the law might result in the denial of a child his natural parents and/or deny natural parents a preemptive right to their children. Now, natural parents can renounce their rights by placing their child up for adoption. But in the former case a natural parent may rescind that renouncement within a specified period of time for the very reason that as natural parents the child is theirs. By law, natural parents have first rights to their children unless they are absolutely unfit. The Court's decision that the Sterns' claims to Baby M overrode Mrs. Whitehead's implies that a contract, any contract, is binding even when it entails overriding claims of natural parents and even when it involves buying and selling human beings.

This brings me to my first and very tentative conclusion. The rights of the natural mother to her child cannot be overridden for the sake of a contract between her and the natural father even what that contract was agreed upon by both parties, because it entails selling a baby, a human being, to another person, and because surrogate parents, in the first instance, do not have prior claims over natural parents. Similarly, a natural father has parallel rights to his child which a contract to buy or sell that child cannot set aside.

Granting this conclusion, however, does not get us very far, because the Baby M case is much more complicated than that. It is more complicated at least in part because while one may grant my contention that a natural parent's rights override the contract in question, the contract in the Baby M case was made between the natural mother *and* the natural father. So while the mother has rights to her child, she also has no right to make a contract to sell the baby in the first place for the very same reasons that as a parent she has rights to her child. Moreover, interestingly, the rights of the natural father, too, to Baby M supercede the contract. As the natural father Mr. Stern has a right to his own baby without having to buy that baby, and at the same time he has no right to enter into an agreement to buy his own baby. The idea of buying (selling) one's own baby is a very strange notion indeed.

The father, Mr. Stern, of course, can argue that he is not buying his baby. He might say that he was merely renting womb space and was the paying the rent. Yet he was doing more than that, because the womb rented happened to be that of the natural mother whom he inseminated. There are actual cases when a woman cannot carry a baby, where a third party is paid or volunteers to carry a fertilized egg, but in the Baby M case the carrier of the baby was also its genetic mother. So the idea of a contract is itself morally questionable not only because (a) a mother cannot sell her baby (nor anyone else's for that matter), and because (b) a father (or anyone else) cannot buy it, but also because, (c) in general, human beings have the very basic right not to be sold (or bought). That the court upheld the contract would seem to be a flaunting of the very basic right of human beings *not* to be sold, a right we have fought for long and hard. One can only hope that the decision will be overturned on those grounds, for the slippery slope precedent to which such a decision leads is not a positive for human rights.

That the contract in the Baby M case is in question, however, does not clear up a second problem. If the natural mother's, the natural father's, and the baby's rights set aside the surrogate contract, are these three equal rights? In the Baby M case Mrs. Whitehead alleged that she had a right to the baby by reason of natural motherhood, and she implied that that right, hers, overrode the right of the natural father to the baby. Although the court disagreed, it is at least clear that at a minimum, in the first instance, the natural mother and the natural father have equal claims to Baby M, albeit for natural and contractual reasons.

Does this lead to the conclusion that the natural mother has *more* in the way of rights to Baby M than the natural father? Yes and no. Traditionally we have upheld a mother's right to her child unless extreme circumstances justified setting aside that right. But there are complications in this case. The baby, Baby M, would never have been conceived in the first unless her mother had contracted to be a surrogate mother and contracted to sell her child. So while Mrs. Whitehead has natural motherhood rights to Baby M, these are not as strong claims as those, say of a nonsurrogate natural mother, since in the case of Baby M, Mrs. Whitehead contracted to have the baby and also contracted to sell it.

At the same time, and by the same sort of reasoning, does the natural father have *more* in the way of rights to Baby M since he contracted to take the baby? This is hardly a sound argument either, because Mr. Stern contracted to buy a baby that was rightfully both his and Mrs. Whitehead's.

The contract, then, is one of the messy sticking points in the problem of surrogate motherhood in Baby M cases. The fallacy of arguing that any such contract is moral or legally binding confuses parental rights with contract rights and threatens both parental rights and the rights of Baby M. Nor can we excuse either Mrs. Whitehead or the natural father for entering into such a contract, because it threatens both their rights as natural parents and the rights of another human being.

The case, however, is even murkier than I have suggested. The court decided to bracket the issue of the contract and argued that

[t]he primary issue to be determined by this litigation is what are the best interests of a child [Baby M] ... Where courts are forced to choose between a parent's rights and a child's welfare, the choice is and must be the child's welfare ... [12]

So the court ruled to decide the case on the grounds of the best interests of Baby M. Traditionally, in our society natural mothers have had prior claims to their children unless there were very good reasons to deny these claims. Traditionally, too, "good reasons" have seldom included economic or even educational ones. The court in the Baby M case, however, questioned that tradition since part of the reason for granting the Sterns Baby M was that the judge found the Sterns more fit than Mrs. Whitehead to provide a good middle class home and education.[13]

Can one justify overriding the natural and certainly traditional mother/child relationship on such utilitarian grounds? The slippery slope of *that* kind of decision is not pleasant to contemplate either. Should mothers on welfare give up their children for adoption to more affluent persons? One expert witness defined a child's best interest as being "1) closeness to be loved, to love and feel nurtured; and 2) a sense of oneness and opportunity to be separate."[14] In the Baby M case the court went further and opted for middle class material values over the value of natural motherhood. While this decision may be merely a reflection of our societal value preferences, nevertheless, it is highly questionable to weigh value preferences of mother/child relationships in cost/benefit terms and to override traditional values of natural parenting for these reasons.

There is yet another argument often cited in defense of the natural father in the Baby M case. The Sterns are good people who cannot bear children of their own. There was no other way for the Sterns to have a child except through surrogate motherhood. Baby M was conceived only because of the Sterns' desire to be parents. She will be loved and cared for as if she was the natural child of both Sterns because of the desire out of which she was conceived. Moreover, good parenting is a virtue, and Baby M's natural father and his wife exhibit more of that virtue than Mrs. Whitehead. Thus however one feels about the legitimacy of the contract between Mrs. Whitehead and the Sterns, if, as the courts argued, the natural father and his wife exhibited the qualities of good parenting and Mrs. Whitehead does not, then the baby should go to the father.

While this may be a good argument in some specific instances, it is often difficult, at best, to evaluate good parenting. Will Mr. Stern and his wife be better parents? They will be richer ones, but better? Mrs. Whitehead was accused of being "manipulative, impulsive and exploitive."[15] She sounds like many normal mothers, a person with cares and feelings. And what are the adjectives that characterize Mrs. Stern? Mrs. Stern has multiple sclerosis. According to one doctor, "Mrs. Stern . . . could be diagnosed as having an adjustment disorder with depressive features."[16] So there is evidence that Mrs. Stern, too, has some human faults.

The question of the welfare of the child brings us to the last stage of the argument — the rights of the baby herself. I have implied that a child has rights — the right not to be contracted for, bought, or sold even to her natural parent. So the root of the problem of surrogate motherhood entails the rights of the child. Baby M situations do not take these rights into account, and indeed, Baby M's rights were set aside both when the contract was made and later when it was upheld by alleging that freedom of contract and rights of surrogate parents take precedence over the the rights of Baby M, and when it was argued that Baby M's best economic interest take precedence over the rights of her natural mother. On utilitarian grounds alone, could one imagine that the benefits of surrogate parenthood, either the benefits to the adoptive parents or the material benefits to the child, could outweigh the emotional damage of a child sold out of motherhood by her own mother to her own father?

Finally, even if the contract under which Baby M was conceived and sold is invalid on a number of grounds, and even if the decision of the court is questionable, what are we to do with those children already born as a result of these agreements and contracts? Barring proof that the natural mother cannot carry out her responsibilities as a mother, a proof that was not demonstrated in the Baby M case, where the natural mother claims her child, Baby M and others like her should be given to that mother.

Footnotes

[1] William Butler Yeats, "The Stolen Child," reprinted in the *New York Times* Letters to the Editor from Javan Kienzle, April 20, 1987.

[2] Adina Schwartz, "Autonomy in the Workplace," in *Just Business*, ed. Tom Regan (New York: Random House, 1984), p. 130.

[3] *Adkins v. Children's Hospital*, 261 U.S. 546 (1923).

[4] *In the Matter of Baby "M", a pseudonym for an actual person*, hereafter referred to as *Baby "M"*. Superior Court of New Jersey, Docket No. FM-25314-86E, unpublished opinion, 93 (1987).

[5] *Lockner v. New York*, 198 U.S. 58 (1905).

[6] See *Adkins v. Children's Hospital* 261 U.S. 546, cited in Schwartz, p. 133.

[7] *West Coast Hotel v. Parrish*, 300 U.S. 379 (1937).

[8] See, for example, Lawrence Tribe, *American Constitutional Law* (Mineola N.Y.: Foundation Press, 1978).

[9] Court, pp. 91-92. See also, Robertson, "Embryos, Families and Procreative Liberty: the Legal Structure of New Reproduction," *Southern California Law Review* 501 (1986).

[10] *Baby "M"*, pp. 91-92. See, again, Robertson, in this regard.

[11] *Baby "M"*, p. 94.

[12] *Baby "M"*, p. 1.

[13] *Baby "M"*, pp. 99-104.

[14] *Baby "M"*, p. 64.

[15] *Baby "M"*, p. 105.

[16] *Baby "M"*, p. 61.

FOR the Legitimacy
of Surrogate Contracts

H. E. BABER

Barring a reversal on appeal, the recent decision concerning the Baby M case establishes the legality of surrogate parenting agreements. The decision is not, however, uncontroversial: many suggest that the practice of surrogate parenting ought not to be legally sanctioned on the grounds that it is immoral. First, it is suggested that no one can acquire a right to any part of another person's body and hence that no contract relinquishing one's biologically based rights over an unborn child to another party can be binding. Secondly, it is argued that the practice of surrogate parenting is detrimental to the interests of the children involved since it constitutes "baby selling." Finally, it is claimed that the practice is exploitative of women, in particular, that it legitimates the exploitation of relatively poor women by economically more advantaged men.

I suggest that none of these arguements are compelling. The practice of surrogate parenting is morally unobjectionable and, indeed, it is typically highly beneficial to all concerned. Further, I suggest that the standard objections to the practice embody unacceptable and empirically unwarranted sexist assumptions.

1. The Right to Control One's Body

Most opponents of surrogate parenting have no objection to the practice of adoption. On the face of it this seems odd: if a woman may relinquish her parental rights over her child after its birth, why may she not do so prior to its birth or, indeed, prior to its conception? Why should we not regard surrogate parent contracts as pre-natal adoption papers?

Some who oppose surrogate parenting arrangements invoke the alleged right of women to "control their own bodies" in support of their claim that women cannot transfer their parental rights prior to birth. The argument is as follows:

(1)   No one can have a right over another person's body or any part of another person's body.

(2)   A fetus is a part of its mother's body.

(3)   Therefore no one but its mother can have any right over it.

(4)   Surrogate parenting contracts purport to confer parental rights over the fetus to other persons.

(5)   Since (by (3)) this cannot be done, all such contracts are null and void.

(1) and (2) are questionable but, even if we grant them under some interpretation or other, (1) is ambiguous. It admits of a strong and weak interpretation because some body parts are, put crudely, detachable and it is unclear whether (1) preludes others from acquiring rights over *detached* body parts. (1), therefore, admits of the following two interpretations:

(1')   There is no time, t, at which one person can have a right over an object which, *at t*, is part of another person's body.

(1")   There is no time, t, at which one person can have a right over an object which, *at any time t'*, is part of another person's body.

(1') is controversial, but even if grant (1'), (1") does not follow. And (1") is implausible: given (2), which is admittedly questionable, it would preclude adoption as well as surrogate parenting. Furthermore, (1') does not preclude my *conferring* a right to a detached body part upon another person prior to its detachment. Even if I cannot *at any time* confer a right-at-t to an item which is a body part at t, it seems that, even at t, I can confer upon another person a right-at-t' to an time which is a body part at t but not at t'. Suppose, for example, I agree to donate blood to you. I sign an agreement giving you a right to my blood once it is drawn. Now given (1') I cannot give you a right to my blood at the time of the agreement, prior to it being drawn: no agreement I make could license you forcibly to draw my blood. Nevertheless, if I agree to donate blood to you then once the blood is drawn you have a right to it, and you acquire that right to it in virtue of the agreement I made while it was still a part of my body. In virtue of this agreement, I have no right to reclaim what was formerly my blood.

This suggests that when it comes to talk about transferring or relinquishing rights we must be careful to distinguish between the time at which the right is transferred and the time at which the recipient acquires the right in question. When I transfer a right to x, then at some time, t, I bring it about the x has a certain right at t', where t and t' may or may not be identical. In light of this consider (4), which we can now see is ambiguous between the following two interpretations:

(4') A surrogate parenting agreement made at t purports to bring it about that another person has the right to an object which is a fetus at t, but not at t', *at t'*.

(4") A surrogate parenting agreement made at t purports to bring about that another person has the right to an object which is fetus at t, but not at t', *at t*.

Now given (1'), only agreements of the sort described in (4") are precluded. Agreements such as those described in (4') are not, and it is (4'), not (4") that in fact seems to convey the burden of current surrogate parenting agreements. Such agreements, though they are made prenatally, confer rights to a child's adoptive parents only *after* its birth and hence are unobjectionable even given (1').

Those of us who oppose abortion would not grant that the fetus is a part of its mother's body, and it does not follow from my objection that it is. My purpose is merely to show that *even if* we regard the fetus as a part of its mother's body and *if*, in addition, we hold that no one can have a right to a *current* part of another person's body, surrogate parenting contracts may still be legitimate and binding. Again, surrogate parenting agreements are typically made prior to conception, before the child who is conceived in fulfillment of the contract is even so much as a body part. No matter. The suggestion is that we must distinguish the times at which rights are transferred and acquired and that a person may enter into an agreement transferring a right to another party prior to the time at which the other party is in the position to acquire that right. I can, for example, give you the right to certain portion of my first crop in exchange for seed money, even though the seed has not yet been planted and, at the time of our agreement, there is not yet anything to which you can acquire rights.

Similarly, it would seem that I can transfer parental rights to a child to you at a time when you are not in any position to acquire such rights, either because the child in question is still, in an extended sense, a part of body or because the child in question does not yet exist. Thus, surrogate parenting agreements cannot be ruled out the grounds that the adoptive parents are not in a position to acquire parental rights to the child involved at the time that the contract is made.

Nevertheless, we still need to consider a range of arguments which turn upon the suggestion that the practice of surrogate parenting is detrimental to the interests of the children involved.

2. Surrogate Parenting is Baby-Selling

Some opponents of surrogate parenting suggest that the practice is detrimental to the interest of babies, who are bought and sold like commondities and otherwise treated as mere means to the ends of their natural and adoptive parents. "Anyone with $10,000," so the objection runs, "can buy a baby."

It should be noted here that currently anyone with functioning reproductive organs and a willing partner can make a baby. Current folk wisdom has it that natural parents, in particular mothers, "bond" with their offspring and are imbued with special intuitions and hormones which guarantee that they will subsequently act in their children's best interests. There is however no empirical evidence to suggest that this in fact occurs either among humans or the higher primates. Similarly, there is no evidence to suggest that adoptive parents who have made a financial investment in their children are more likely to regard them as mere possessions or to mistreat them than are biological parents. Thus there seems to be no compelling consequentialist reason to suggest that it is very much in the interest of children to be raised by their natural parents.

There is not compelling non-consequential reason to reject surrogate parenting arrangements either. Opponents of the practice suggest that it is unacceptable because the children who are conceived in accordance with surrogate parenting agreements are conceived as mere means to further their mothers' self-interested ends. Nevertheless, quite apart from surrogate parenting arrangement, children are frequently conceived as means to their parents ulterior ends. Women get pregnant in order to bully reluctant partners into matrimony and to shore up faltering marriages; men beget children in order to carry on their family names and prove their virility. And both men and women have children in order to surround themselves with families and to provide themselves with security in old age, to perpetuate themselves, after a fashion, and to further a variety of other fundamentally self-interested ends which they cannot adequately articulate. Indeed, it would be metaphysically odd to conceive a child for *its* sake -- presumably to confer the benefits of actuality on a being hovering in a Meinongian netherworld of unactualized possibilia.

In fact, most babies are conceived for their parents' sakes, to further their various ends. If conceiving a child as a means to some further end is morally wrong then most cases in which children are conceived, even quite apart from any surrogate parenting arrangements, would be morally objectionable on this account. But most such cases are not morally objectionable hence conceiving a child to further some ulterior end is not *per se* morally wrong. If it is not morally wrong to conceive a child to further some ulterior end, then conceiving a child in fulfillment of a surrogate parenting contract is not on these grounds objectionable. Now it may be suggested that even if conceiving a child for some ulterior end is not in and of itself wrong, conceiving a child for certain purposes is morally questionable. Nevertheless it is hard to see why conceiving a child to fulfill a surrogate parenting agreement is more objectionable than, e.g. having children in order to provide security for oneself in old age, which is a common practice and which most people regard as morally unobjectionable.

Thus, there is no compelling reason to believe that surrogate parenting agreements are contrary to the interests of the children involved. It remains to be seen however whether surrogate parenting arrangements are contrary to the interests of the women who act as surrogate mothers.

3. The Practice of Surrogate Parenting Exploits Women

Prima facie it would seem that surrogate parenting agreements benefit all the adults involved. Through a voluntary agreement an infertile couple gets a child and its surrogate mother gets a substantial sum of money, in most cases, more than she could otherwise earn for nine months work, for nothing more than the "work" of having a baby. It is argued however that surrogate parenting arrangements are exploitative and thus against the interests of the women who act as surrogates.

Surrogate mothers, it is argued, are compelled by their relative poverty and by their powerlessness as women in a sexist society to sell their services to richer, more powerful males. This, it is suggested, is exploitation and exploitative practices are not morally acceptable.

Now, as a preliminary to determining whether surrogate parenting arrangements are exploitative it is crucial to get clear about what exploitation is. It may be suggested that any arrangement in which a relatively poor, relatively powerless person sells goods or services to a richer, more powerful one is fundamentally exploitative insofar as any such arrangement is one which exploits the relatively less desirable situation of one party. Someone who understands exploitation this broadly however does not have an objection to surrogate parenting arrangements: his quarrel is with capitalism as such. While his objection may be well-taken, our purpose here is not to assess the moral acceptability of the capitalist system. Rather, we want to determine whether the surrogate parenting arrangements are morally unacceptable in a way that other transactions in which goods and services are exchanged are not. Thus we assume, for the sake of the argument, that not all such transactions are exploitative. Our purpose is to elucidate the conditions which render some exchanges of goods or services exploitative and hence morally unacceptable.

A paradigm case of exploitation is the Biblical story of Esau who, on the verge of starvation, sold his birthright to his younger brother, Jacob, for a bowl of pottage. Three features of the story are significant. First, Esau's situation was abnormally bad: it was a predicament from which we would expect that any "minimally decent Samaritan" with food to spare would extricate him without demanding any payment.

Secondly, the price which Jacob paid for Esau's birthright was unfair: Esau's inheritance was by any reasonable standards worth considerably more than a bowl of pottage. Finally, we assume that Esau would never have exchanged a bowl of pottage for his patrimony if his situation were not abnormally bad. These elements of the Biblical narrative point to three conditions which, in general, appear to be individually necessary and jointly sufficient for a transaction's being exploitative. Arguably, an exchange of goods or services is exploitative if and only if the following conditions are met:

(1)   The situation of the seller must be one which would be recognized by him and members of his community as, in some sense, abnormally bad.

(2)   The price which the buyer pays must be substantially less than the value of the goods or services he procures.

(3)   If the seller had not been in an abnormally bad situation he would not have sold his goods or services for the price offered by the buyer.

These conditions require further explication. We would want to know, for example, what constitutes an *abnormally* bad situation, what community's standards figure in determining when such a situation obtains, how the value of goods and services is to be determined and so on. Nevertheless, it seems that on some reasonable interpretation these are the conditions which make a transaction exploitative. Furthermore, it does not seem that, on any reasonable interpretation, these conditions obtain universally in surrogate parenting transactions, indeed, it is quite clear that they did not obtain in the transaction which occasioned the Baby M case.

Clearly, the first condition did not obtain. The Whiteheads, a single-income, working class family, were much less well off financially than the Sterns but the financial situation of Mrs. Whitehead, the surrogate mother, was scarcely abnormally bad. Indeed, when their case came to court the Whiteheads were prepared to prove that they were able to provide adequately for Baby M. In addition, there is no reason to think that Mrs. Whitehead's situation was abnormally bad in any other respect. Furthermore, it is not clear that the second condition was met either. Mrs. Whitehead earned $10,000 for nine month's "work" as a surrogate mother. As a female high school drop-out with no recent work experience and no skills it is unlikely that she could have earned as much for any other service she was qualified to provide. Certainly, it seems morally repugnant to put any price on a human life. But the question is not whether Baby M was worth $10,000; the question is rather whether Mrs. Whitehead's services were worth that sum, and when we consider what these services consisted in, it seems that $10,000 was, if anything, generous. Conceiving a child and carrying it to term is not skilled work: no special education or training is required. It is not especially hazardous. And it imposes far fewer constraints on a person's liberty than virtually any other job available: apart from occasional doctor's appointments, tests, and the actual birth, Mrs. Whitehead was free to go about her business, a benefit that most women in the labor force, chained to typewriters from 9 to 5, should envy.

Nevertheless, one might ask, if the prospects of surrogate mothers are so rosy, why the widespread sense that women who enter into surrogate parenting arrangements are exploited? I suggest that it is because many people greatly overestimate the intensity of the attachment which women feel toward their unborn or newborn children and, indeed, the frequency with any such attachment occurs. If women universally formed intense "bonds" with their babies prior to birth or shortly thereafter, so that giving up a baby to be raised by someone else would inevitably be an emotionally devastating experience, then one might expect that only women who were in truly desperate straits would agree to act as surrogate mothers. Furthermore, in such circumstances, if we were to regard the payments to surrogate mothers not as fees for services rendered but rather as compensation for emotional distress then the case might be made that $10,000 was negligible when compared to the amount of distress surrogate mothers typically endured. Thus, if all women "bonded" to their babies prior to birth or shortly thereafter and, as a consequence suffered extreme and lasting distress if compelled to give them up to be raised by others, there would be good reason to believe that surrogate parenting arrangements were exploitative.

There is however no evidence to suggest that all or most mothers do in fact "bond" to their babies or that those who give up their babies shortly after birth suffer extreme or long-lasting distress. The current popular literature does indeed encourage pregnant women to cultivate relationships with their unborn babies and enlightened hospital routine now includes a quiet time with baby shortly after birth to facilitate "bonding." In addition, there are many people who very much want to believe that women bond to their babies since many people have a vested interest in believing that women are very different from men psychologically and emotionally, that these differences are innate, and that they include a much greater stake in matter related to reproduction and child rearing. Conservatives who wish to maintain traditional sex roles are included in this group but so are new style feminists who reject the old, liberal assimilationist ideal, and, indeed, so are a great many decent, undogmatic people without any axes to grind who are simply frightened by the changes in the role of women which have occurred in the past ten or fifteen years.

The will to believe is a potent force, and given the widespread desire to believe in "bonding" it is possible to believe in the teeth of substantial empirical evidence to the contrary. Thus, just prior to the decision in the Baby M case a (female) commentator on *60 Minutes* commended Mrs. Whitehead for fighting to keep her baby in contrast to the hundreds of surrogate mothers before her who had "repressed their natural maternal instincts." Nevertheless there is no reason to believe that this extremely ill-defined instinct exists either among humans or among the higher primates. And if, in fact, there is no reason to think that most women who act as surrogate mothers "bond" to their babies and suffer extreme emotional distress when they must relinquish them, there is no compelling reason to regard surrogate parenting arrangements as exploitative.

4. Conclusion

I have argued that the practice of surrogate parenting is not ordinarily contrary to the interests of either the women who act as surrogate mothers or to the children involved and hence that the practice is morally acceptable. Naturally, like agreements of any kind, surrogate parenting contracts may involve fraud or exploitation. This is, however, a good reason to make surrogate parenting contracts legally binding: by legalizing a practice we allow for the possiblity of regulation and secure the protection for the law for all parties concerned.

Biographical Note

My arguments are sound and stand on their own merits: in general, biographical considerations about the arguer should play no role in our assessment of an argument. For those who believe otherwise and for the merely curious, however, I should like to point out that as I write this I am seven months pregnant with my third child.

Why a Surrogate Mother Should Have the Right to Change her Mind
A Feminist Analysis of the Changes in Motherhood Today

BARBARA HILKERT ANDOLSEN

The "Baby M" trial is a compelling drama. One reason why this case arouses such strong reactions is that it raises disturbing questions about the meaning of motherhood. Furthermore, it raises them at a time when the social definition of motherhood is in transition. In order to appreciate more fully the debate about values provoked by this case, it is helpful to situate the case within the context of changes in social understandings of motherhood.

Motherhood as a Social Institution

Since human beings are profoundly historical beings, all moral judgments take place within a particular historical context. It is especially important to realize that decisions about surrogate motherhood[1] occur within a specific historical situation, because there is a dangerously misleading tendency to describe motherhood as a natural function which remains essentially stable throughout history.

The dominant cultural image of motherhood which we have inherited in current society is a product of the Industrial Revolution. The Industrial Revolution separated the workplace from the home. It stripped the homemaker of many productive functions and isolated many mothers at home with their young children. Such women were compensated for their loss of other functions with an ideology of motherhood extolling the social influence which women wielded through shaping the characters of their children, particularly their sons.

Strong elements of racial/ethnic and class bias are frequently implicit in the dominant social image of motherhood. It is a bitter irony, for example, that poor black women have too often worked long hours caring for white offspring, while separated from their own children.[2] Throughout much of the nineteenth and twentieth centuries, it was predominantly white women from the middle and upper classes who were the "ideal" mothers devoted entirely to the care of their children.

Those mothers became increasingly isolated in the home throughout most of the day. Fathers were "at work"; many single female relatives also worked outside the home; older children were in school. It became harder for middle-class families to find servants. A growing number of mothers could no longer share child care with members of an extended family. Thus, many mothers took almost total responsibility for child rearing.

Child development experts created theories of child rearing which reflected the new situation in which mothers were left with almost sole responsibility for young children's well-being. These experts not only mirrored the new mother-child isolation, they also justified and idealized it.[3] Theorists of child development -- some of whose work was widely disseminated in popular culture -- emphasized the crucial importance of early childhood experiences which were increasingly under the control of the mother. A close, exclusive relationship between mother and child was described as both natural and necessary for the healthy development of the child. Child development experts frequently established "scientific" standards for child care wich exhibited ethnic, racial and class biases.

The portrait of the good mother as one who is in the private home focusing her energies on the healthy physical and mental development of her child was the product of a certain set of historical circumstances. However, those circumstances have been changing. Since the start of industrialization, some women have followed "work" into the factory and office. First, single women, then women with older children entered the workplace. Most recently, women with small children have chosen to go out to work. By 1985, half of all women with children *under three* held paying jobs. At first, married black women were more likely to be in the paid labor force. Now their white counterparts have joined them in more nearly equal percentages.

Moreover, there has been a reversal in the relationship between class and employment for women. In the nineteenth century, it was predominantly married women [white] from the middle and upper classes who devoted themselves to husband, children, and home. Poorer women, disproportionately drawn from black and immigrant groups, were forced to supplement meager family incomes through (poorly) paid labor. Today, women from the middle and upper classes have career opportunities which make paid employment very attractive. It is more likely to be the poor (or working-class) young woman who has children early and, perhaps, remains at home with those children. With limited marketable skills, such a woman may well prefer homemaking to the tedious, insecure, low paying jobs available to her.

Mary Beth Whitehead and Elizabeth Stern are typical of this reversal. Whitehead, who is currently a full-time homemaker, dropped out of high school. Her work history in low paying service jobs is episodic; she also collected welfare for a time. Stern has two doctoral degrees and worked consistently in professional positions until the custody dispute over Baby M. It is, perhaps, a measure of our cultural ambivalence about working mothers, as well as a reflection of the Sterns' child rearing preferences, that, when Dr. Stern was under scrutiny as a mother, she took a leave of absence from her job and planned to return to work only part-time.

The Baby M case challenges us to examine our views about the meaning of motherhood at a time when our understandings of mothers are in flux. This case forces us to reexamine our notions about the relationship between motherhood and caring, rational control, and autonomous choice.

A. Trustworthy Care

1. Maternal Love

The Baby M case touches a hunger for trustworthy human caring. Since at least the late eighteenth century, women in general -- and mothers in particular -- have been the cultural icons of reliable human love. However, as women's roles in society change and as fewer women devote themselves exclusively to the caretaking functions of wife and mother, our notions about dependable nurture are shaken. Part of the controversy about whether Mary Beth Whitehead should retain custody of Baby M springs from assumptions about a "natural," loving, mother-child bond which may seem one of the few remaining vestiges of trustworthy care in an otherwise impersonal, materialistic, and individualistic society.

We have idealized the care provided by (middle class, white) mothers isolated with their children in private homes. When mothers and children are socially isolated, the mother becomes the almost exclusive source of continuity, care, nurture and tenderness for children. As Adrienne Rich proclaims, the needs of the child become "vaster than any *single* human being could satisfy, except by loving continuously, unconditionally, from dawn to dark, and often in the middle of the night."[4] The cultural ideal of motherhood seems to offer a guarantee of continuous, unconditional love even in the middle of the night.

We may be led to wrong conclusions about surrogate motherhood, if we mistake a cultural ideal of mother love shaped by a particular set of historical circumstances for evidence of an immutable, instinctive love between birth mother and baby. During a recent discussion about the Baby M case, one attorney made just such an assumption. He proposed that there should be a clear legal presumption that the woman who gives birth to a child is its mother.[5] He argued that legal rights should remain with the birth mother for the sake of the child. He reasoned that a child needs stable care and asserted that our one reliable source of care was our biological mothers.

The maternal bond between a birth mother and child is a far more complex phenomenon than that attorney recognized. Indeed, arguments which postulate an instinctive maternal love raise larger questions: are there some innate female values, or are women socially conditioned to display certain distinctive virtues? Posed as an either/or, these questions lead us into a trap of opposing nature/body to history/culture. Such a trap is especially dangerous to women who have been oppressed by identifying them in a unique way with nature and the body and by denying them an opportunity to be active agents in history and creative shapers of culture. Women, like men, are *both* bodily beings immersed in nature *and* historical beings whose understandings of their bodies and their relationships with the rest of nature have a history and are shaped by culture.

Pregnancy, childbirth, and lactation are bodily experiences. They may give rise to a physiologically-based form of maternal attachment. However, the expression of that bond (if such a bond exists) is highly influenced by the material and cultural circumstances in which mothers and children find themselves. Among human beings, love is not an instinctual response. It is a moral virtue -- one whose acquistion and maintenance is influenced by social and historical conditions. For example, historical records from the first half of the eighteenth century in France are filled with accounts of mothers from a range of economic classes who sent their newborns away to be cared for by wet nurses for long periods without apparent compunctions. The women who served as wet nurses frequently provided grossly inadequate care; infant mortality rates were very high. Yet, there is little evidence that the biological mothers' reproached themselves for failure to fulfill their maternal obligations to their children.[6]

Whatever the bonding which takes place between gestational mother and child during pregnancy and childbirth, their relationship is culturally malleable. Thus, Mary Beth Whitehead and some of her supporters make a highly dubious assertion when they claim that she should have custody of Baby M because, as the child's gestational mother, she has a unique biologically-based ability to nurture Baby M.

Ironically, at the same time that the Baby M case evokes notions of a maternal instinct somehow rooted in the very physiological process of pregnancy and childbrith, it also reveals a profound distrust of women's nurturing skills. The isolation and idealization of the mother and child in the home have resulted in the scapegoating of mothers for every perceived failing in their children. Mary Beth Whitehead was criticized by one expert because she offered her baby daughter stuffed animals to play with instead of pots and pans; he also alleged that Whitehead played patty cake improperly. Such intense scrutiny of Mary Beth Whitehead's mothering techniques was only a particularly brutal example of the constant criticisms voiced about contemporary women's child rearing methods. William Stern, the baby's father, was not subject to such searching scrutiny for fitness as a parent.

2. Fathers and Care

If the Baby M case challenges us to reexamine our understandings of motherhood, it also requires us to investigate afresh the cultural meanings assigned to fatherhood. The meanings of fatherhood have also changed throughout history. In some ways, industrialization has deprived fatherhood of cultural weight. Industrialization removed fathers'contact with their children for long hours each day. "Physically absent the whole day, tired out in the evenings, the father did not have any great opportunity to develop a relationship with the child [especially the young child who might be asleep by the time the father returned home.]"[7] During the nineteenth century, social change reduced the role of father to that of an economic provider and, perhaps, an occasional playmate or adviser. To the extent that society acknowledged a role for fathers in nurturing their children, that role was clearly secondary to the role accorded the mother.

In recent decades, the advent of a new wave of feminism coupled with the movement of many [white] mothers into the labor force has led to a reconsideration of the role of fathers. Many women are demanding that father assume a greater responsibility for the nurturing of their children. Fathers are being told that they have an obligation, along with mothers, to provide tender, continuing care (even in the middle of the night). According to his own testimony and reports of experts, William Stern stands ready and eager to provide care for his daughter. William Stern's willingness to assume the obligations of fatherhood gives him a strong claim to custody. Along with Mary Gordon, I do not believe that it is just "to discount William Stern's claim, or automatically to devalue it because he did not bear the child in his body."[8]

B. Rational

The Baby M case arises in a society in which, to a extent perhaps unprecedented in history, women and men experience becoming parents as a choice legitimately subject to their rational control. Most women believe that it is both possible and morally desirable to control the reproductive powers of their own bodies. Women's attempts to control their own fertility are not new in human history. As ethicist Beverly Harrison recounts:

Even under the most adverse conditions, women as a group have attempted to develop some controls in relation to their fertility -- in every culture, without exception, regardless of existing morality or religion. But women's lack of social power, in all recorded history, has made this effort to control fertility difficult for a great many, probably most. Many women have managed to do whatever seemed possible, given available knowledge, to avoid too-numerous pregnancies.[9]

Although we know even less about the struggle of some women to *assist*, not prevent, fertility, it seems plausible that some women have also managed to do whatever was possible, given available knowledge, to achieve strongly desired pregnancies.

In the United States today, many women experience an unprecedented degree of success in preventing unwanted births. For many women, reliable means of contraception are available -- as are safe, elective abortions.[10] Moreover, many women assert that such control of reproduction is a moral good. They insist that sexually active women should be able to choose whether or not to become a mother and how to harmonize the timing and demands of motherhood with other responsiblities and commitments in their lives.

Over the last two decades, large segments of American society have accepted this notion that human beings have a right to control their reproductive processes. This new attitude tends to create a corollary. The notion of a right to prevent unwanted parenthood broadens into a notion of *a right to experience wanted parenthood*. However, human control of bodily fertility has proved more intractable than the more simplistic notions of "reproductive choice" indicate.

A large number of American couples have found that they are unable to conceive a child through normal coitus. Estimates indicate that as many as one in five couples experiences involuntary infertility. Infertility confronts individuals with the limits of their capacity to control their bodies. For some middle and upper-class couples, this lack of rational control may be especially frustrating. As one woman experiencing fertility problems explained: "In my life, if I wanted something, I'd figure out how to get it, and go out and get it. Now here's something I have no control over. And no matter how hard I try, there's nothing I can do"[11] Human beings cannot always bend their bodies to fit their plans for life.

I am not suggesting that human intervention in the reproductive process is morally wrong per se. We have an obligation to use our initiative and intelligence to further human well-being. Enabling women and men who would otherwise be childless to satisfy their desire to become parents is one way to further human well-being, as long as the techniques used do not exploit or seriously injure others. Women and men must make *responsible* use of the techniques available to channel procreative powers.

Techniques which involve the use of another woman's body to carry the desperately wanted child are unusually problematic from an ethical perspective. Because of the dignity of the human person as a body/self, special moral caution should be exercised in any situation in which one person proposes to use another person's body as an instrument to achieve the first party's aims. The moral risk of seeing another human being in purely instrumental terms is revealed in the language of one "expert" report filed in this case. "In both structural and functional terms, Mr. and Mrs. Stern's role as parents to Baby M was achieved by *a surrogate uterus and not a surrogate mother.*"[12] Does surrogate motherhood inevitably deprive a woman of her human dignity by reducing her to a useful uterus? Or is it possible to structure surrogate motherhood relationships in such a way that the gestational mother is not treated solely as a means to achieve the infertile couples' dreams? If the latter is possible, what conditions would be necessary to protect the human dignity of the gestational mother?

The possiblity of hiring a surrogate also raises troubling questions about harm done to other persons within a very tangled web of relationships. Will the child born of a surrogate relationship suffer undue adverse consequences? Many surrogate mothers have already borne other children. What is the impact on these other children who participate in the surrogate's pregnancy only to see a sibling be given to another household? What about the responses of the surrogate's sexual partner, if she has one? What is the impact of this choice on members of the surrogate's extended family?

C. Choice

Increased control over human reproduction means that a growing number of women and men experience the conception and birth of a child as matters of choice. The spreading practice of surrogate motherhood means some women have yet another choice. They may choose to conceive and to carry a child whom they intend to surrender at birth to the biological father. Over the past 10 years, 500 women have chosen to become surrogate mothers.

For Judge Sorkow a crucial issue in the Baby M case was Mary Beth Whitehead's legal (and moral) responsibility to honor a surrogacy contract which she had *voluntarily chosen* to sign. He described Whitehead as having reneged on her promise and as seeking to avoid her obligations. The judge rejected the argument that Whitehead should not have been asked, in advance of the birth, to give irrevocable consent to relinquish custody of the child. He dismissed suggestions that there should be a waiting period after the birth of a child during which a surrogate mother could withdraw from the agreement to surrender the child.[13] Sorkow argued that Whitehead, unlike a birth mother surrendering a child for adoption, made her decision before she experienced the stress of pregnancy. She had time to consider her choice and to seek advice. She was free to negotiate the terms of the agreement and did request and receive some small changes. According to the judge, once she had accepted the terms of the contract and conceived William Stern's child, Whitehead was obligated to carry through with her promise to surrender the child to the Sterns.

1. The Fickle Surrogate Mother

There are some feminists who argue that, once a woman chooses to enter into a surrogate contract, ther terms of the contract should be binding and the woman should be obligated to surrender the child as promised. For some of these feminists, any proposal that surrogate mothers should be allowed to change their minds and keep their babies is an especially distasteful one. Such feminists are reluctant to do anything which might promote the stereotype that women are fickle, flighty, or incapable of making up their minds. Some feminists are afraid a legally guaranteed waiting period would suggest that women are less able to act as reliable decision makers. Such a policy would, they contend, reinforce the notion, deeply embedded in Western culture, that women are too weak minded to make morally trustworthy choices.

There is another potentially disturbing aspect of Mary Beth Whitehead's change of mind. She decided not to surrender her baby in part because of bodily experiences. She gave birth; she saw her newborn baby; she breast fed the infant. These physical events were among the factors that led Whitehead to conclude that she would not give her baby up to William and Elizabeth Stern. Again, Whitehead's behavior seems to confirm misogynist western cultural traditions. Women's perceived deeper ties to their bodies have been used as the rationale for disqualifying women as moral agents. According to one highly influential cultural tradition in the West, women are less capable of that abstract, "disembodied," rational judgment which is the hallmark of ethical wisdom.

Admittedly, Whitehead's change of mind evokes all the cultural stereotypes about fickle, untrustworthy women. However, the solution to this threat to women's standing as moral agents is not to insist that birth mothers be compelled to honor the contractual promises which they made prior to birth. Society should not legalize surrogate arrangements which designate the child as the legal offspring of the contracting wife at the time of birth.

Rather, feminists and others need to challenge the view that "disembodied," rational judgment is the moral ideal. It is time to insist that "all our knowledge, including our moral knowledge, is body-mediated knowledge,"[14] It is out of *diverse* embodied experiences that human beings begin to sort out conflicting moral claims. Moreover, decent regard for other human beings means that we must strive to take their bodily experiences into account when balancing moral claims. It is not clear to me whether any society can define the terms of a surrogate mother arrangement in a fashion consistent with respect for the human dignity of all the parties involved. However, I propose that any morally acceptable policy to regulate surrogate contracts would have to include a provision guaranteeing a period of time after birth in which the surrogate could reconsider her decision to surrender the child. The process of pregnancy and childbirth -- with all its physical impacts and its varied cultural meanings -- is a very complex one. I suggest that no woman, even one who has borne a child before, can give knowledgeable consent in advance to surrender her newborn. I make this recommendation even though it entails a regrettable uncertainty and a potentially devastating disappointment for a couple which may have already endured the sorrows of infertility.

2. Choice in a Free Market

The section of the Baby M decision which discusses the surrogate contract relies on liberal philosophical assumptions about autonomous individuals who exercise radically free choice when entering into contracts. A laissez-faire, free market model seems to be the backdrop for the judge's decision. But Mary Beth Whitehead was not simply a free agent in a free market. She was an economically embattled woman. While Whitehead does not appear to have been motivated primarily by a desire for money, she and her husband were in precarious economic circumstances. They had filed for bankruptcy in 1983; and, at the time of Baby M case, they were in default on two mortgages on their home and were facing foreclosure proceedings.

Judge Sorkow dismisses the relevance of the economic circumstances of the parties to a surrogacy contract. His sympathy for infertile couples feeling the pangs of an intense drive to procreate apparently mollifies any concern about possible exploitation of lower-income women as childbearers for relatively wealthy couples. Sorkow argues that neither party has an undue advantage, since the surrogate's economic vulnerability is balanced by the emotional vulnerability of the infertile couple.

I argue, to the contrary, that the economic disparities in this and similar arrangements cannot be easily dismissed. There is a tremendous disparity between the economic resources of the Whiteheads and the Sterns. The emotional vulnerability of a couple desperately seeking a child they cannot produce from their own union should not be overlooked. However, in this case the Sterns' desire for a child did not simply put them on a par with the Whiteheads in a private arrangement between the two couples. Rather, the Sterns' longing for a baby made them vulnerable to manipulation by a third party, Noel Keane of the Infertility Center of New York. Keane charged $10,000 for arranging the surrogate relationship.[15] In 1986, Keane's surrogate practice grossed $600,000[16] The potential for economic exploitation of *both* the surrogate mother and the infertile couple is grave. In England, such payments to agencies which serve as brokers for surrogate contracts have been made illegal. Legislation outlawing similar profit making agenices should be given serious consideration in the United States.

3. An Unnecessary Choice?

Many couples who choose to contract with a surrogate mother do so because the wife is infertile. Surrogate motherhood is one in a severely constrained range of reproductive choices for such a couples. An examination of some causes of infertility suggests that we could prevent infertility, in at least some cases, thus limiting the number of couples considering the choices to employ a surrogate.

It is commonly thought that women who delay child bearing -- often because of social barriers to combining parenthood with a career -- face higher risks of infertility. While Elizabeth Stern is not absolutely infertile, the Sterns were in an analogous situation. Their choices about reproduction were limited by a social situation in which childbearing is unnecessarily difficult to reconcile with educational and career responsibilities. The Sterns delayed having children in the early years of their marriage. During those years, Dr. Stern faced very heavy educational and professional demands, which, the couple felt, would not allow her to care adequately for a child. By the time the Sterns had reached a point where they could take on the responsbilities of parenthood, Elizabeth Stern had discovered that she suffered from multiple sclerosis. If medical school and residency programs were flexibly designed to accommodate family needs, the Sterns would have had a realistic option to have a child early in their marriage, before Dr. Stern's medical problems were diagnosed; and the Baby M case might never have arisen.[17]

Some infertility problems emerge, because a woman faces career pressures which lead her to delay childbearing until it is too late. Involuntary female infertility may also result from damage to the reproductive system casued by sexually transmitted diseases. It can also be caused by exposure to workplace hazards that imperil fertility. "No one knows how often workers suffer miscarriage or infertility due to chemicals in the workplace, ...but in 1985 the Federal Centers for Disease Control called human reproductive failure a 'widespread and serious' problem, and one of the ten most prevalent work-related diseases."[18] There are social policies such as improved sexual education programs, increased funds for research on sexually transmitted diseases, tighter enforcement of occupational safety and health laws, increased availability of high quality day care facilities, or mandatory parental leave programs which would "eliminate" infertility problems for many couples without recourse to the use of surrogates.

Concluding Remarks

Cultural notions of motherhood based on the isolation of mother and children in the private home of the industrial era are being challenged. This transformation confronts us with the realization that bodily human experiences, including the experiences of pregnancy, childbirth, and the nurture of young children are always understood through culture and history. The Baby M case is one more occasion which confronts us all with the need to clarify contemporary concepts of maternal and paternal obligation.

Availability of reliable contraceptives and of safe, elective abortion have led women and men to expect to exercise effective control over whether and when to have children. Greater reproductive control is one more cultural factor that leads many of us to grant a high priority to the values of rational control and autonomous choice when faced with decisions about reproduction. However, as a result of increased rates of involuntary infertility, large number of women and men are painfully confronted with the limits of human control over their reproductive destinies. It is urgent that we evaluate decisions regarding surrogate motherhood asking whether such arrangements are consistent with the dignity of all the persons involved. We should strive to insure that some (often economically vulnerable) women are not reduced to the status of merely useful uteri in order to gestate the children ardently desired by others. It is especially important to explore social policies which would prevent avoidable infertility and, hence, to minimize the need to resort to surrogate motherhood.

Footnotes

[1] Surrogate mother is a rather unsatisfactory term for several reasons. The parties in a surrogate mother arrangement do not intend that the surrogate will be the female who nurtures the child; and, in that sense, the surrogate is not a mother. However, in this case and in most surrogate arrangements apparently, the woman who provides the service both conceives and bears the child. From a biological perspective, therefore, she is simply the mother, not a "surrogate" mother. In spite of these linguistic difficulties, I will use the commonly accepted term.

[2] While there are fewer dometic servants in the home today, day care centers where many of the workers are racial/ethnic women are a new variation on this older them.

[3] Ann Dally, *Inventing Motherhood: the Consequences of an Ideal* (New York: Schocken Books, 1982), p. 10.

[4] Adrienne Rich, *Of Woman Born: Motherhood as Experience and Institution* (New York: Bantam Books, 1976), p. 4, emphasis mine.

[5] This is in contrast to some legislative proposals which would recognize the "infertile" female party in a surrogate contract as the legal mother from the time of birth.

[6] Elisabeth Badinter, *The Myth of Motherhood: An Historical View of the Maternal Instinct* (London: Souvenir Press [E & A] Ltd., 1981.

[7] Badinter, *Myth of Motherhood*, p. 258.

[8] Mary Gordon, " 'Baby M' -- New Questions About Biology and Destiny," *Ms.*, June, 1987, p.26

[9] Beverly Wildung Harrison, *Our Right to Choose: Toward a New Ethic of Abortion* (Boston: Beacon Press, 1983), pp. 155-56.

[10] Adolescent women may have difficulty in gaining access to either birth control or abortion services; poor women may have difficulty paying for abortions.

[11] Sue Woodman, "Crazy for a Baby: What Happens to Women in the Grip of the Infertility Cult?" *New York Woman*, November/December, 1986, p. 142.

[12] Robert Hanley, "A Reporter's Notebook: Tactics in Baby M Trial," *New York Times*, February 9, 1987, B3.

[13] Proponents for such a waiting period frequently draw an analogy to the waiting period granted to birth mothers who surrender a newborn baby to strangers for adoption.

[14] Beverly Harrison, *Making the Connections: Essays in Feminist Social Ethics*, edited by Carol S. Robb (Boston: Beacon Press, 1985), p. 13.

[15] This is in addition to the $10,000 to be paid Mary Beth Whitehead, if she bore and surrendered a full term infant to the Sterns.

[16] Anne Taylor Fleming, "Our Fascination with Baby M," *New York Times Magazine*, March 29, 1987, p. 35.

[17] At the time when Elizabeth Stern decided to forego childbearing, a woman with multiple sclerosis who carried a pregnancy to term was thought to be at increased risk of results, such as paralysis, vision impairment or loss of hearing. Current medical opinion holds that there is only a remote possibility that pregnancy and childbirth would have worsened Dr. Stern's condition. Therefore, if she had borne a child early in her marriage, Elizabeth Stern might well have had both a baby and reasonably good health.

[18] Carol Marshall, "Fetal Protection Policies; An Excuse for Workplace Hazard," *The Nation*, April 25, 1987, p.532.

"All Birthing Should Be Paid Labor" — A Marxist Analysis of the Commodification of Motherhood

JANE OLLENBURGER AND JOHN HAMLIN*

Surrogate mothering can be viewed from a number of perspectives. In this paper we utilize a socialist feminist framework to pinpoint some critical issues and indicate crucial implications. We believe that a socialist feminist perspective, one which seeks to clarify the workings of patriarchal capitalism by explicitly focusing on the exploitation of women, will add a new dimension to the issue of surrogate mothering.[1]

Socialist Feminism

The marketing of infants and children is a social phenomenon which has existed for thousands of years. In contemporary western nations, adopting children often carries a rather stiff price tag. The current custody case involving Baby M adds a different dimension to the production of children for sale. Putting the Baby M case into socialist feminist perspective allows us to draw attention to the changing role of motherhood.[2] No longer does the adage "flag, motherhood, and apple pie" refer to sacred social symbols. Motherhood has been exposed for what it has always been under capitalism, albeit in latent form, a commodity; with babies becoming increments of surplus value.

According to the Marxian theory, a commodity by definition possesses two contradictory moments in an antagonistic relationship (Marx 1976 [1867]). A commodity must have use value, that is, must

---

This project was a joint project of equal effort. The order of names does not indicate level of participation.

* *Special thanks to: Judy Gillespie, Georgia Keeney, J. Clark Laundergan, and Tim Roufs for reviewing an earlier version of this paper.*

have utility for someone. But having utility is not enough to transform something into a commodity. A thing must also have exchange value; it must be something for which others are willing to trade. The commodity possesses a dialectical character. For the utility (use value) to be realized it must be exchanged; once exchanged it becomes a thing to be consumed or used, not a commodity, for its exchange value no longer exists.

Under capitalism labor itself becomes a commodity to be bought and sold in the marketplace much the same as all other commodities. The basic difference, and a very critical difference, is that labor produces value. Labor is exploited in the marketplace precisely because it is capable of producing *more* value than was paid for the original commodity of labor power. Within capitalism a process of proletarianization takes place, eventually separating people into two antagonistic classes, the bourgeoisie owners of the means of production and the proletariat laboring class; in consequence, one class, the proletariat, will swell in number.

Since Marx paid little attention to the gender division of labor, he neglected some critical differences within the working class. To begin with, women labor in the paid work force along side men. The gender division of labor has operated to reinforce patriarchal divisions to the benefit of capital and men (Young 1981). Therefore, women can be identified as surplus labor or a reserve army of labor to be maneuvered around the labor market as needed. Second, women have labored in the unpaid labor market of home and voluntary associations with little or no formal recognition or monetary benefits. This aids capitalism as workers (both men and women) are reproduced on a daily basis to toil in the factories and offices across the faceless landscape of capitalism. Women also literally reproduce the labor force through childbirth. In this role of unpaid labor, women have been doubly exploited in as much as women have produced use values critical for the maintenance of patriarchial capitalism, but the product has been deemed valueless because it lacked exchange value.

It can be argued that motherhood through the institution of marriage, has always been an exchange relationship. But the purpose has been one of solidifying social relationships between various clans and tribes (Levi-Strauss 1966: 109). The exchange was different in kind than the exchange of other goods because the outcome of motherhood produced children as well as vital social connections, while the exchange of other goods only produced social connections.

The Baby M case provides an opportunity to look at the interplay of gender, class and issues critical to women of color, all of which are significant components of a socialist feminist perspective. Each of these social factors in surrogate mothering will be viewed within this framework; first, however, we must briefly describe the case.

The Case of Baby M

Baby M, now named Melissa Elizabeth Stern, was over a year old before she received her name as it was awarded by Judge Sorkow in a New Jersey court. Although the case was specifically a battle between two families, it is readily generalizable since it represents a continuing manifestation of class conflict.

The Sterns are a classic bourgeoisie "yuppie" family, or in current terms, a "dink" (dual income no kids). William Stern, aged 40, holds a doctorate in biochemistry, earns approximately $43,000 a year and is Jewish. He wanted a child because he felt compelled to continue his family bloodlines since, according to his lawyer, his father and mother are deceased, having died in the United States, and all other living relatives were killed during the Holocaust. Elizabeth Stern, aged 41, holds a doctorate in human genetics and is currently a pediatrician, earning about $48,000 a year as an assistant professor of pediatrics at the Albert Einstein College of Medicine in New York. She initially delayed having a family until she was finished with her medical residency in 1981. A symptom associated with multiple sclerosis was first discovered in 1972, eventually leading to medical attention in 1979. Then, in late 1982, she decided based on that diagnosis that preganancy would potentially worsen the disease, and elected not to bear children. The Sterns decided to try surrogacy.

The Sterns contacted the Infertility Center of New York, a business which, for a fee, brings together potential surrogates with potential parents. The fee includes $10,000 to the agency, an additional $10,000 to the surrogate plus an estimated $5,000 in expenses. Therefore, for a

$25,000 fee the Sterns would receive an infant produced from Mr. Stern's sperm and another woman's egg. The Sterns viewed 300 applicants and eventually chose Mary Beth Whitehead.

Mary Beth Whitehead is a housewife, aged 29, who is married to Richard Whitehead, aged 37, a sanitation worker who earns about $28,000 a year. Mary Beth was sixth of eight children of a schoolteacher and a beautician. She did not finish high school, married at age 16, and had two children by her 19th birthday. Her two children are Ryan, 12, and Tuesday, 10. The Whiteheads chose to have no more children. Mary Beth Whitehead sort of "looks like" Elizabeth Stern, a reason she was chosen as the surrogate. She also wanted to be a surrogate to give to others "the gift of life and the joys of parenthood."

However, after Baby M was born Mary Beth Whitehead decided she could not surrender the baby and refused to sign over custody. She declined the $10,000 fee and took the child from the Sterns. The Sterns obtained a court order to have the baby returned and over a year passed before the baby was legally named and officially adopted by the Sterns.

Class, Gender and Women of Color: Issues in Surrogacy

The state, as represented by the court, explicitly described the class backgrounds of the parties involved in the Baby M decision. The court, in justifying these lengthy descriptions, claimed it was serving the best interests of the child. In serving the "best interests of the child" social class will always play a predominate role since lower class families cannot offer the material comforts of upper-middle class families; standards of love, care and general well-being will therefore be measured with upper-middle class criteria.

The court description of the class differences between the Sterns and the Whiteheads clearly show that the court favored the Stern family. William Stern's father was a banker until they were forced to leave their homeland. William worked to help support the family once in the United States. William went on to college and attended graduate school at the University of Michigan in biochemistry. Elizabeth Stern's father was a biochemist at Michigan State University. She attented graduate school at the University of Michigan and received her doctorate in human genetics. The Sterns postponed having children while Mrs. Stern attended Medical School and completed her residency. The court noted that the family placed a great emphasis on education, as demonstrated by their professional upper-middle class lifestyle. They were also represented as being deeply religious. Mrs. Stern's father was a lay reader for a church, and they were married by a minister friend of the family. Mr. Stern's family had been persecuted in Germany for being Jewish. The emphasis on education clearly represented class values, as did the focus on the level of religious participation. One more point is critical: when Mr. Stern's mother died, William Stern became the only family survivor, thus if the family name was to be carried on a child needed to be produced. The description of the Stern's background rendered by the court was all very positive.

The Sterns' background is not unlike other upper-middle class families nor is the Whiteheads' background atypical of lower working class families. Mary Beth Whitehead dropped out of school at age 15 and started working part time jobs. She married Richard Whitehead at age 16; at the time he was 24. Richard Whitehead had been honorably discharged from the army in 1971. They had two children, and since they did not want any more he had a vasectomy. The stability of this family contrasts with the Sterns precisely in the ways that the two classes contrast. The Whiteheads changed residences frequently, 12 times in 8 years, often staying with family members. They were separated for a short period during which time Mary Beth collected public assistance, a not uncommon survival strategy for lower class families. They reunited after this short separation. In 1983 they were forced to declare bankruptcy. The court emphasized that Richard Whitehead drifted between jobs and unemployment, holding 7 different jobs in 13 years. He has maintained his current job, however, since 1981. The court neglected to recognize the influence of the overall labor market on job insecurity, particularly as it impacts lower class families. The mid-to late 70's were a time of high unemployment and recession. The court also noted that Richard Whitehead is an alcohol abuser; according to the middle class standards of the courts, Mr. Whitehead drinks too much. The court did not take into account the fact that many "problems" associated with Mr. Whitehead are shared by other Viet Nam veterans. In contrast to the description of the Sterns, the court description of the Whiteheads focused on negative attributes rather than positive ones.

In family court, where the standard is the best interest of the child, that interest will be stated and measured using middle class rules. If lower class women are to have their labor protected as well as their rights as mothers, then legal contracts must be clearly spelled out and binding. To address this issue more fully it is necessary to consider specifically gender issues, especially as we consider the impact of patriarchy and classism on this type of court decision.

Is it possible to define the Baby M case in purely gender terms? The answer is yes. Mr. Stern is the sole survivor of his family. He could adopt a child but there appear to be many obstacles blocking the path. If the genetic pool is to be maintained he must use his sperm to impregnate the egg to produce "his" baby.

In the legal contract set up for surrogate reproduction, the advantage clearly goes to the male. This includes control over the surrogate's personal habits since, by contract, she may not smoke, take drugs, drink alcohol during pregnancy, or have sexual intercourse during the period around insemination. Violation of these conditions would be considered a breach of contract. She is diligently screened for biological and pyschological abnormalities. However, the contracting couples are often not screened beyond a verification of their bank balances. But the control the male has extends even further. If the woman is in danger she may choose to abort the child, but at no other time does she have that power over her own body. The power of abortion is controlled by the male. Via the legal contract, the woman signs away the right to control her body; yet the partriarchal classist courts claim the contract to be invalid if it is not in the "best interests of the child." Therefore, she will never have the control unless she can negotiate a valid contract.

When looking at the interaction of patriarchy and classism, the issue of women of color cannot be ignored. Women of color are not likely candidates for practicing surrogate mothering. The demands for the product, white children, and thus the demands for the producer of surplus value, are not something over which a minority will have control. The demand for white able-bodied infants is a reflection of our racist society. For most minority women surrogating will be a non-issue. However, it could be an issue from the point of view that upper class male control of the process of child production will further segment the labor market, creating a group of chronically unemployed minority women in highly industrialized countries. This will not be the issue in peripheral countries where minority women work labor intensive, low paying jobs and make up about 80% of assembly line workers. However, it is possible for third world women to become targets for baby producing with potentially less capital outlay costs and fewer legal difficulties for corporate surrogate enterprises.

Volunteerism/Charity v. Paid Employment

One of the issues which arose from the Baby M controversy is whether or not surrogacy is an act of charity or is it, in fact, paid labor. The surrogates themselves often justify their choice by making a claim of volunteerism "talking about what they describe as the ultimate act of charity" (*Newsweek* April 13, 1987: 23). Yet, social opinion clearly views the money as an important component. While 20% of the people in a survey sympathized with the surrogate mother, only 8% felt she should have been given the baby (*U.S. News & World Report* April 13, 1987: 60), as one woman stated "I feel sorry for [Whitehead] for having to go through it, but on the other hand, she got paid" (*U.S. News & World Report* April 13, 1987: 60). Throughout the language of the trial and in the news coverage we read about the surrogates "volunteering" their services. "Whitehead, 30, a New Jersey housewife, *volunteered* her services to the Infertility Center of New York last year because, she said, she wanted to help a childless couple" (*Time* Sept. 22, 1986). Surrogates "volunteer" their services, yet are paid $10,000 plus expenses.

Legislative concerns also appear to focus on the volunteer/ paid employment issue. New York is a case in point. Of the estimated 500 babies born through surrogate arrangements in the past ten years, 100 have been born in New York State. This has prompted proposed legislation to restrict surrogacy. More significant than the legislation itself are the reasons behind the bills being proposed. "The restrictions are justified, the report by the State Senate Judiciary Committee argues, to guard against a concern that underlies much of the public debate over surrogate parenthood. It is the fear that, left unchecked, some women may choose surrogates as a matter of convenience, to avoid delaying a career with a pregnancy or because they fear that a pregnancy would make their bodies unattractive" (*NYT* Jan. 31, 1957: L30). Or as suggested in *Time*, there is a fear of women ". . . among the poor, turning to careers as professional breeders" (Jan. 19, 1987: 58).

It appears that the Baby M case cuts to the core of patriarchal capitalism by illuminating the inherent contradiction between the fundamental nature of patriarchy (domination of women) and the fundamental nature of capitalism (exploitation of labor). The commodification of motherhood would help to undermine the insipid nature of patriarchy and expose the 'callous cash nexus' of patriarchal capitalism. It would appear that law and the media's expression of public opinion are oriented toward maintaining male control of women's reproductive capabilities.

Although in a more perfect society volunteerism would be desirable as a general practice, given the vast inequalities of our society and the importance of occupation in establishing identity, all work should be paid and recognized as worthy of pay. Surrogacy should be no different. Since the late 1800's the issue has been the inverse for women: how do you get men to take responsibility for babies they father? When children were considered an asset to the family economically, whether in agrarian societies or during early capitalism when child labor was encouraged, men were often given custody of children (Brown 1981). With the rise of monopoly capitalism from 1880-1920 (also known as the progressive era) children came to be defined as liabilities and women were granted custody. There has been enough volunteer motherhood.

Contract v. Custody

In deciding the case, Judge Harvey Sorkow claimed the overriding weight of the evidence for the decision was based on the best interests of the child: " . . . when conflicts arose the 'best interests of the child' should prevail. Thus it was her best interests, and not the existence of a contract, that led him to award custody of Baby M to Stern" (*Time* April 13, 1987).

Contracts, like unions, can provide protection for the laboring classes. Here the "best interests of the child" become defined as middle class interests. One ethics expert, Lisa Newton, from Fairfield University in Connecticut, claims that Baby M should not be judged under contract law but should be treated as "custody cases — in which the better parents win"(*U.S. News & World Report* Jan. 19, 1987: 15). Clearly the "better parents" is often synonymous with the wealthier parents. Therefore, it is imperative that contracts be treated as binding legal documents and not as simply a guideline for surrogacy. Disputes should be settled on the basis of contract law and not family court.

However, there is a definite patriarchal advantage in the way contracts currently read. Women who wish to be surrogates need to have representation in the formation of the contract. Also, escape clauses are vital to maintaining the mother's control over her own body. An escape clause would allow the surrogates a limited time after they give birth to change their minds. Although opponents claim that allowing women to change their minds would destroy surrogacy, the only thing it truly might damage is the profit margin. Valid contracts would protect working class women from exploitation by upper class men and women in the commodity production process, and the escape clause would protect women from the patriarchal control of men.

Women will need special safeguards built into the agreement to insure that wages are sufficient and work conditions satisfactory. Technical legal language has historically been a tool used by powerful members of the white patriarchal system in exploiting working class women and women of color. Contracts need to be as jargon free as possible, using both languages in bilingual cases.

Conclusion

The commodification of motherhood raises many questions and issues that must be addressed with a high degree of seriousness. However, many questions will not even be considered until surrogacy becomes commonplace. Women will have to question on a personal level the contradiction between cultural definitions of mothering and bonding, and the realities of commodity production. Alienation is always a problem in commodity production and there is good reason to believe that, given traditional ideology surrounding mothers, alienation could be even more severe in the surrogacy labor process.

The dynamic tension between capitalism and patriarchy has resulted in years of latent exploitation, trapping women within families. This represents the control of men over women generally and over reproduction more specifically. Women labored and produced children (surplus value) and were virtually unpaid for their efforts. Surrogate mothering brings this masked exploitation to the forefront and exposes non-paid baby production for what it is in capitalist society — naked commodity production.

Exploiting one's capacity to labor is unjust because it provides an increment of value for which one was not paid. Now women produce a laborer for sale, the increment of surplus value is potentially immense. Class, gender and women of color divisions combine to create new forms of exploitation. Upper-middle and upper class families can buy babies; lower-middle and, in some cases, lower class women can sell babies.

However, socialist feminists should support surrogate mothering precisely because it does provide payment for labor that exists and until now has gone unpaid. The more capitalism's exploitative nature is exposed, the higher the likelihood its tranformation. We would go so far as to say that all birthing should be paid labor, as should all aspects of the housework and family maintenance.

Marx saw the transformation of labor into commodities as the last and most important change necessary for the development of capitalism. He also thought that a mode of production would not disappear until all the productive forces within it had developed. According to Engels (1972: 71-72) production is in both things and people, although he pursued that idea in family form rather than specifically motherhood. Perhaps we are witnessing a new direction in the development of productive and reproductive forces. What we have thought about in terms of producing material things has only been half of capitalism's productive capabilities; producing the laboring classes has been the other half. When both producing material goods and services and reproducing the labor force are developed to their fullest potential under capitalism, social transformation can take place.

Notes

1. Information concerning the Baby M case comes from the *New York Times, Time, U.S. News & World Report, Newsweek,* the official court opinion.

2. There are many sources one could consult for a fuller description of socialist feminism. A couple of good sources are: *Women and Revolution: A Discussion of the Unhappy Marriage of Marxism and Feminism.* 1981. Edited by Linda Sargent. Boston: South End Press; *Thinking about Women: Sociological and Feminist Perspectives.* 1983. Margaret L. Andersen. New York: Macmillan; *Feminist Frameworks: Alternative Theoretical Accounts of the Relations Between Women and Men. 1984. A. Jaggar and P.R. Struhl. New York: McGraw-Hill.*

References

Brown, Carol.   1981. "Mothers, Fathers, and Children: From Private to Public Patriarchy. Pp. 239-267 in Lydia Sargent (ed.) *Women and Revolution: A Discussion of the Unhappy Marriage of Marxism and Feminism.* Boston: South End Press.

Engels, Frederick.   1978 [1942]. *The Origin of the Family, Private and Property and the State.* New York: International Publishers.

Levi-Strauss, Claude.   1966. *The Savage Mind.* Chicago: University of Chicago Press.

Marx, Karl.   1976 [1867]. *Capital Vol. One.* New York: Vintage.

New York Times.   Jan. 1, 1987 — March 31, 1987.

Newsweek.   Sept. 1, 1986; p. 66.
        April 13, 1987; pp. 22-23.

Superior Court of New Jersey Chancery Division/ Family Part, Bergen County. March 31, 1987. *In the Matter of Baby "M",* *a pseudonym for an actual person.*

Time. Sept. 22, 1986; p. 36.
Jan. 19, 1987; pp.56-58.
April 6, 1987; p. 88.
April 13, 1987; p. 71.

U.S. News & World Report. Jan. 19, 1987; p. 15.
April 13, 1987; pp. 60-61

Young, Iris. 1981. "Beyond the Unhappy Marriage: A Critique of the Dual Systems Theory;" pp. 43-69 in Lydia Sargent (ed.) *Women and Revolution: A Discussion of the Unhappy Marriage of Marxism and Feminism.* Boston: South End Press.

A Cross Cultural Analysis of Several Forms of Parenting
Mother, Genitrix, and Mater

MICHAEL R. HILL

-- *"The issue here is not so much technological as sociological."*

Herbert Brail, attorney

-- *"Even an infant needs her own space."*

Harvey Sorkow, judge

Introduction
Private Troubles and Public Issues

Melissa Stern was born March 27, 1986, in New Jersey. For one so young, she has experienced or been the subject of interstate flight and fugitive hegira, legal battles involving her own court-appointed attorney, social controversy, the voracious attention of an insensitive media industry, and a place in history as the famous Baby "M". Judge Sorkow (1987: 26-27), in his opinion awarding custody of Melissa to her genetic father and terminating all parental rights of her genetic mother, notes professional evaluations indicating Melissa to be a "a mellow, alert, easy-to-care-for child who is blessed with a 'sunniness of disposition that is a delight to see.' " She is also "a curious and social baby and adjusts to her strangers and social situtations easily." One hopes these resilient character traits flower as Melissa matures and discovers the intricacies in which her personal biography has become inextricably enmeshed in the public issues of American social conflict. The following analysis is offered with a view to explicating the interconnected personal troubles and public issues now drifting toward yet another reconsideration of a primary American social institution: family. This blatantly sociological enterprise has its own role to serve in the reflexive and hopefully emancipatory hermeneutic of social change (Giddens, 1987a, 1987b), but it is also hoped that this analysis will at some future time make at least some sense to Melissa herself.

Confronting distinctly personal troubles is by no means a unique experience in this society. Many of us, in the process of maturation, have acquired a substantial cache of guilty secrets, unresolved conflicts, desperate hopes, doubts, injustices, frustrations, betrayals, and stupidly bungled projects. We are often prime architects of our foibles, but at times we play the unwitting if not unwilling dupe to the deceptive fabrications, insanities, and insensitivities of friends and fellows who abuse our trust (Goffman, 1974/1986). These private troubles are the existential stuff of life in human society as it is now organized. Much that Melissa Stern has encountered and will continue to meet are personal troubles that only she can recognize, pick her way through, and presumably resolve with dignity and growth.

Melissa's life journey began in the private troubles of her father, William Stern, and his wife, Elizabeth Stern. The Sterns wanted to raise a family (hardly a nefarious project in this intensely familistic society), but discovered that Elizabeth Stern's incipient (and hopefully mild) multiple sclerosis made pregnancy an unacceptable risk. Discouraged by their exploratory inquiries concerning adoption, the Sterns eventually learned about and investigated the possibility of surrogate reproduction. The consummation of a surrogate reproduction contract between William Stern, Mary Beth Whitehead, and her husband, Richard Whitehead, led to Mary Beth's artificial insemination with William's sperm and the subsequent birth of a baby girl, now known as Melissa Stern. As part of this arrangement, William agreed to pay $10,000 to Mary Beth who in turn agreed to sever her parental rights where the newborn baby was concerned.

Had this plan gone as proposed (as hundreds of similar arrangements in fact have), Melissa's troubles would have been much reduced. Instead, Melissa's mother, Mary Beth Whitehead, became enmeshed in unforeseen personal troubles of her own. Among others, she decided to retain her parental rights and to raise the baby girl within her own family. These events set the stage for a deeply emotional drama in which two sets of legally incompatible personal troubles, those of William Stern and Mary Beth Whitehead, collided head on resulting in Melissa's well-chronicled odyssey. A vortex of personal troubles, claims and counterclaims ensued, entangling not only Melissa and her genetic parents, but also Elizabeth Stern, Richard Whitehead, the Whitehead's two children, Melissa's maternal grandparents, and friends of both families. Were this the full story, however, Harvey Sorkow's (1987) juridical resolution of these troubles would not have made front page headlines in national newspapers (see, for example, Hanley, 1987a, 1987b; *New York Times*, 1987; Shipp, 1987).

The private troubles of the assembled litigants and concerned parties became a catalyst wherein several public issues surfaced, became inflamed, and developed lives of their own which have nothing whatever to do with the happiness and well-being of Melissa, the little girl with the sunny disposition. Thus, we encounter here an unusually cataclysmic intersection of public issues and private troubles. Whereas Melissa must eventually come to grips with the notoriety of her own biography, she will do well to recognize that neither she nor her parents created the public issues that catapulted her into the history books. Her multiple parents only tried to resolve their own private troubles in their own ways. It was only later that they -- and the rest of us -- discovered that their private troubles were shared by many -- and could potentially be shared by a quite significant portion of our society. As Mills (1959) helps us understand, the personal troubles of the Sterns and the Whiteheads resonated in a loud, dissonant chorus echoing the public issues of a capitalist, patriarchal, and familistic society.

Sociological Imagination and Family

The myriad public issues finding voice in Judge Sorkow's New Jersey courtroom are rooted in our most enduring social patterns, including: family, law, religion, politics, partriarchy, racism, capitalism, and class. In this chapter, I concentrate on issues related to family. There is a tendency when investigating or thinking about matters related to these patterns to reify them, to conceptualize them as essentially immutable, fundamental, intrinsic, unquestionable. Understanding the actual map of our social world in this taken-for-granted, everday sense is in itself a tall and difficult project requiring intellectual discipline and sensitivity (Giddens, 1987a; Goffman, 1974/1986; Deegan and Hill, 1987; Mead, 1934; Reinharz, 1979/1984; Rubin, 1976; Schutz, 1971; Taft, 1915/1987). Comprehending that our taken-for-granted institutions often assume radically different forms than posessed -- or recognized -- at present requires a degree of insight and reflexivity possessed by few people, including sociologists. With this in mind, Giddens (1978a, 1987b) argues for the practical necessity of adopting "the sociological imagination so eloquently outlined by the distinguished American sociologist, C. Wright Mills (1959). If we fail to critically examine history, anthropology, and alternative futures as Mills and Giddens advocate, we run the almost certain risk of entrapping ourselves in reifications, ethnocentrism, and political impotence.

Most commentators agree that surrogate reproduction is intimately linked to the institution of "family". Failure to adopt historical and anthropological sensitivities, however, leads to strange, ethnocentric pronouncements about presumed universal aspects of family and parenting. Sensitive social scientists help us avoid such mistakes. Julia Kristeva (1974/1986), for example, provides a deep, texturally complex analysis of the meanings of motherhood and family in Chinese and western societies. Even within the restricted orbit of the industrialized countries of the contemporary world, however, history reveals a range of family forms and child rearing practices (Poster, 1978) that would cause many narrow-minded, self-righteous defenders of mythically invariant family morality to retreat in embarrassment, hopefully with apologies for their insensitive bigotry. Jessie Bernard (1972/1982) demonstrated the surprisingly varied ways in which modern Americans arrange themselves in conjugal groupings of greater and lesser duration and commitment, including: traditional marriage, communes, cooperatives, one-night stands, swinging, intimate networks, households of unrelated individuals, serial polygamy, geriatric marriage, *menage à trois*, group marriage, companionate celibacy, and feminist households. Add to this list the variations devised by gays and lesbians and the permutations are formidable. Human beings invent, experiment, and adapt, often with vigor, grace, good humor and commitment. They also bungle, cheat, and hurt each other, but this is not new. There are some who simply and unreflexively lump this diversity and playfulness under the rubric of "sin", but these are people who lack a sociological imagination -- to say the least. The best critical evidence leaves us with what is to some a startling conclusion: there is no such thing as *the* natural family form. We give life to many family forms, all as natural as the next, some enjoying greater or lesser popularity at different times and among various subgroups in western societies.

The image of the "ideal" independent conjugal nuclear family (husband, wife, and their jointly produced genetic children) has been powerfully projected as *the* family as though this form is more "natural" or legitimate than any other possible arrangement. The reasons why this particular familial pattern has received massive ideological approval in American society lie beyond the scope of this chapter, but interested readers will find a good introduction to several fundamental public issues in Barrett and McIntosh (1982). The point here is that discussions of surrogate reproduction get caught in needlessly convoluted distortions and serious conceptual mistakes if their authors assume from the outset that there is really only one kind of legitimate and natural family form.

Multiple Parenting

A cross-cultural perspective on the forms of parenthood lets Melissa Stern rationally locate herself in a matrix of multiple parents. On examination, we see that multiple parentage is quite common, even among families who believe themselves to be model examples of the independent conjugal nuclear type. The possibilities for multiple parenting are not new, but they have been augmented by recent developments in bio-techno-medical research (cryogenics, gene splitting, *in vitro* fertilization and embryo transfer, especially). One thing needs to be said, however: that the surrogate reproductive procedures (artificial insemination) resulting ultimately in Melissa's birth are exceptionally low-tech and do not depend intrinsically on medical intervention. Indeed, were it not for the cultural mores of the reproductive partners in surrogacy arrangements, impregnation could be readily achieved through normal coition. Whereas genuine and serious concerns are raised by the high-tech reproductive technologies, these concerns, insofar as they are generated by technology *per se*, do not apply to surrogate reproduction of the type which brought Melissa into this world.

Given the disparate variations in marriage and parenting found trans-historically worldwide, it makes sense anthropologically to speak of *forms* of parenthood. These general patterns, three each for mothers and fathers, are outlined in Table 1. The forms of fatherhood, for example, can all be filled by one person. This result is assumed in the "ideal" independent conjugal nuclear family. The husband is the genetic father. As genitor, he nurtures and sustains his wife during her pregnancy. Finally, in the role of pater, he helps rear and socialize the young child. Thus, if we mistakenly assume that the independent conjugal nuclear family is the only natural family form, we are likely to erroneously conflate the various forms of fatherhood.

If we take a broad view, as the sociological imagination suggests we should, we find that fatherhood roles in some cultures are distributed over a large number of people. While only one male can technically be the genetic father, some biologically naive and promiscuous groups believe and act upon the idea that it is possible for a woman to be the genetic father. Sustenance during pregnancy can be accomplished by several males, and is sometimes required in a somewhat unusual -- to contemporary occidental ears -- variation in societies where it is believed that the fetus will grow only if the mother has coitus on a frequent basis with several males during pregnancy. The presumption is that the seminal fluid nourishes the fetus. It is this relatively rare belief and practice from which the term "genitor" derives, but support of the mother and her fetus certainly includes many possibilities other than coital service. Additional forms of nurture can be easily identified and provided by a wide range of persons. These include emotional resources, financial aid, medical assistance, and birthing preparation. Finally, following the child's nativity, the newborn may be raised by yet another father, or even by a group of men who share equally or hierarchically in the pater role.

TABLE 1: Forms of Parenthood

MALE　　　　　　　　　　　　FEMALE

Genetic Father
  (contributes sperm)

Genitor
  (provides supportive
  environment for
  pregnant
  genitrix)

Pater
  (provides care and
  socialization of child

Genetic Mother
  (contributes egg)

Genitrix
  (provides gestation
  and/or supportive
  environment for
  pregnant genitrix)

Mater
  (provides care and
  socialization of child)

* * * *

By analogy, a similar analysis is possible for motherhood. The roles of genetic mother, genitrix, and mater are all filled by the wife in the "ideal" conjugal nuclear family. *In vitro* fertilization, however, makes it possible to clearly separate these three roles. For example, an egg supplied by one woman (genetic mother) is fertilized and implanted in a second (genitrix), with the resulting child raised by a third (mater). These roles are also open to cooperative arrangements. For example, nurturing a pregnant woman can be shared, thus expanding the role of genitrix to non-pregnant but supportive women. Finally, any number of women can be designated or seek to be maters, taking responsibility for the care and socialization of the newborn.

Looking at parenthood in this way absolves Melissa from unnecessary confusion and fruitless questions such as "Who are my *real* parents?" In reality, she has multiple parents who have clearly identifiable roles, all essential to Melissa's conception, gestation, birth, and subsequent well being. All her parents have made *real* contributions. One the male side, her genetic father is William Stern, her genitors are William Stern (who paid the medical bills) and

Richard Whitehead (who saw his wife through her pregnancy), and her pater is now William Stern (assuming that Judge Sorkow's custody decision is not reversed or significantly modified). On the female side, her genetic mother and genitrix is Mary Beth Whitehead. The court record indicates that Elizabeth Stern, herself a physician, participated in an ancillary genitrix role by giving emotional reinforcement and medical advice. Her primary mater will be Elizabeth Stern (and may include Mary Beth Whitehead in a secondary mater role if subsequent courts allow visitation). This accounting of Melissa's various parents appears bizarre only if one applies the unique and anthropologically strange case of the "ideal" independent conjugal nuclear family as one's point of reference.

In fact, such multiple parent situations are not at all unusual. They are commonly found in families involving death of a spouse and subsequent remarriage by the survivor; in families dissolved and reassembled through the increasingly common practice of serial polygamy; and in families formed by adoption and foster parenting. Surrogate reproduction adds no new twists to parenting roles already in place and socially accepted.

Parenting: Ideology and Praxis

Our concepts of family and parenthood are changing, but sometimes we let obvious, easily assimilated changes slip away unnoticed when our rhetoric becomes intemperate and ethnocentric. We forget that the "ideal" independent conjugal nuclear family is, in fact, far from common in practice when we look closely at the parenting roles in American society. With high rates of teenage promiscuity and pregnancy, not to mention multiple-partner sexual liasons among adults both married and single, it is reasonable to conclude that in significantly increasing number of pregnancies there is no congruence between the genetic father and the genitor/pater in many so-called "ideal" marriages. Without a court test and paternity evidence provided to the contrary, the vast majority in this society are quite happy to assume and act as though the husband in a conjugal nuclear family is necessarily the genetic father of his children, even when a quick calculation of the odds could easily lead to alternate conclusions.

When we reflect comprehensively on the ways in which parenting roles are currently distributed in American society, the ideological hypocrisy that conflates parenting praxis with the "ideal" independent conjugal nuclear family quickly crumbles. For example, participants in popular prenatal birthing programs often utilize someone other than the genetic father to fill the genitor/genetrix role as "coach" for breathing exercises. Courts appoint guardians to represent the interests of unborn children, a legal institutionalization of the genitor/genitrix role. Many children find themselves paired to multiple maters and paters (and fictive kin) through the widespread practice of appointing godparents in religious rituals. I leave untouched the various roles adopted by grandparents, some having sued successfully in court to establish visitation with their grandchildren.

Bitterly contested custody suits attending divorce create unfortunate acrimony and sorrow, but reasonably amicable custody resolutions appear much more the norm. Our society is readily and easily legitimating remarriages wherein wives and husbands frequently become maters and paters to children where others (often faceless unknowns, sometimes not) fulfilled the role of genetic parent as well as genitor or genitrix. The growing number of single parent families (of several types) calls for a pragmatic redefinition of "family" and parenting roles. This call is increasingly hard to ignore. Expanding day care service widens opportunities for more men and women of the community to participate in the pater and mater role (in addition to traditional pater/mater niches such as school teaching, scout leadership, and Big Brother/Big Sister programs). We must account also for the *in loco parentis* responsibilities of boarding schools and colleges, the roles of nannies, wetnurses, baby sitters, and others who act as mater and pater on intermittant as well as regular bases. In short, although the concept of parenthood in this society is frequently conflated with the ideological ideal of the independent conjugal nuclear family, we generally act quite differently, routinely splitting parenthood roles and assigning their performance to a surprisingly wide variety of individuals. There is a conceptual gap between what we say we believe parenthood to be and what we actually take-for-granted and act upon where parenting is concerned.

There are some who would blindly ban the distribution of parenting roles that accompany surrogate reproduction. Such proposals are authored by unthinking critics who do not see that precisely the same distributions can be accomplished by misadventure using fully legitimated routes. Consider this hypothetical example: A man and woman marry, but subsequently discover that the woman cannot have children. Family, friends, and neighbors whisper in guarded tones, "My, my what a shame, he would make such a good father." The couple tries to redefine their childlessness as a positive opportunity for interpersonal growth, but they are told they are "selfish" to think that way. Family and friends, however, continually remind the couple of their "disappointment" and "tragedy". Succumbing to self-doubt and other pressures, the marriage ends as the couple is unable to conceptualize a meaningful future. The man quickly remarries, but not wisely. A child is born of this new union, a child who almost immediately becomes the subject of a bitter custody challenge and the center of rancorous divorce proceedings in which the man eventually agrees to pay $10,000 in alimony as a move to "get his manipulative new wife off his back." In light of documented circumstances which throw reasonable doubt on the ability of the mother to provide a nurturant and stable home, the court awards custody of the child to the man, a not uncommon event in this day and age. Time passes. Eventually, the man and his first wife begin dating again and discover to their mutual delight that they hadn't really given marriage a chance. They remarry and the woman eventually adopts the child as her own. Were this a movie script, would we not feel pangs of sympathy, at least for the child who has found a happy home in the midst of an otherwise troubled and imperfect world? I think so. And if we can, then I think we can feel ever so much better about Melissa and her new life with the Sterns, a life that the Sterns wanted, planned, and presumably prayed for.

I do not assert that the above hypothetical case and the surrogate reproduction arrangement entered by William Stern and the Whiteheads are in any way similar in terms of *intent*. But, I do argue that the resulting parenthood roles and many of the structural conditions are remarkably congruent. Society already provides a fully legitimated sequence of events that has much the same result as surrogate reproduction by simply resorting to a variation on serial polygamy. Indeed, were surrogate reproduction to be outlawed, as some propose, I suspect it would not be long before persons would collude to purposefully implement a moderately complicated three-stage scenario (marriage-divorce/second marriage-pregnancy-divorce-custody & alimony settlement/remarriage-adoption) in much the same way that many couples a few years ago routinely divorced and remarried annually in order to gain federal tax benefits based on marital status. Human beings are remarkably inventive and resourceful when push come to shove. It is mistaken to think that simply outlawing a practice means, in our insititutionally redundant bureaucratic society, that it cannot be accomplished legally by other fully legitimate, socially acceptable procedures.

Legislation and Emancipatory Futures

It is wise to be wary when male-dominated legal, medical, and political professions dip their collective hands in any till where large sums of public and private funds are freely flowing and the interests of newborn babies are at stake. With regard to surrogacy, thoughtful people have raised several issues of concern (see, for example, Brail, 1987; *Harvard Law Review*, 1986; Hollinger, 1985; Katz, 1986; Mellown, 1985; Sorkow, 1987), but most nonetheless see a role for surrogacy in specifiable circumstances. Avi Katz (1986), for example, in a paper awarded the Columbia Law Women's Association Prize, meticulously puts to rest the false equation of surrogacy with baby selling and reviews the efficacy of various approaches to surrogacy legislation. These analysts are of one voice in calling for legislative guidance to institutionalize equity for all parties involved in surrogate reproduction.

Writing and enacting legislation is a social project, one which defines, enables, and limits human action. Present laws become frameworks within future humans (some like ourselves, and some no doubt quite different — at least in their values) will reproduce, raise families, and even marry. Thoughtful legislation in a democratic society creates opportunities for emancipatory alternative futures which may be at present beyond our ken. Articulating such futures is one of the main tasks of sociology (Giddens, 1987a, 1987b; Hill, 1984; Mills, 1959). These futures are the critical and political produce of active sociological imagination.

Caution is advised such that we do not ethnocentrically, too quickly, or unnecessarily, bar socially and personally beneficial avenues to life, liberty, and happiness. Legislative action requires anthropological, historical, and critical sensibilites in order to strike an equitable and emancipatory balance between public policies and personal interests. Emancipatory social consciousness calls forth self-determination, mutual understanding and public cooperation (Mead, 1934; Taft, 1915/1987). I hope these goals will be uppermost in the minds of legislators who draft and vote on bills designed to regulate surrogacy. Legislation encouraging cooperative social consciousness and structurally supporting its realization can only be applauded. It is certain that surrogacy statutes will be enacted. I urge here that, whatever else is accomplished by codification, we not run roughshod over the emancipatory potentials called forth by hundreds of people who, in resolving their private troubles, have given life to surrogacy as a focus of public issues. At the least, these issues include the following: upward mobility, feminist sisterhood, inter-class solidarity, ethnic and communal legacies, and renewed sensitivity to the needs and status of orphans.

Upward Mobility: Much has been made in sensational popular accounts concerning the relatively large, lump-sum fees paid to surrogate mothers. Before uncritically dismissing these payments to the genetic mother/genitrix as exploitive, there is another dimension to be explored, one in which these sums play an enabling, constructive, emancipatory role. Opportunities for working-class women to gather substantial sums of money at one place within a constrained time period in this society are virtually non-existent. Critics who would bar these women and their families from financial resources that could easily purchase a major life-dream (a habitable home, needed surgery, a child's college education, and so on), should more closely examine their own class biases. A careful reading of Rubin's (1976) brilliant exploration of life in working-class families will help sensitize even the most complacent middle-class pundit. If we are serious about class leveling and upward mobility, then we should be cautious about shutting the door on equitably reimbursed surrogacy arrangements between freely consenting parties.

I do not know what the Whiteheads plan to do with the surrogacy fee paid by the Sterns, that is their own private trouble. Given the special origin of the money, attendant as it is on Melissa's birth, one hopes it might be dedicated to a constructive project found especially meaningful by the Whiteheads. Melissa Stern should be encouraged to feel joy insofar as the familial desire that brought her into this world not only gave delight to William and Elizabeth Stern but also resulted in a rare, beneficent material opportunity for the family of Mary Beth and Richard Whitehead.

Sad to say, a professor I know recently expounded venomously that, "Surrogate mothers only want to see their babies grow up in comfortable upper middle-class home!" Presumably, I and others in his audience were supposed to think this goal unconscionable. A black woman sitting nearby was heard to say in a loud stage whisper, "It sure beats living in the ghetto!" I concur. Families, with full social approval, have long used marriage as a mechanism for upward mobility. Impoverished mothers have routinely given up their genetic children to adopting maters and paters, "So the kids could have a better chance at life." To impugn identical motivations when they surface in the hearts of multiple parents freely engaged in surrogate reproduction is not equitable. That we have such gross material inequality, that is the unconscionable reality, one that *is* a genuine public issue (Scott, 1984). Given that barbarous inequality is the order of the day, can we blame people who want something better for their genetic offspring, if not for themselves? The prospects for Melissa's material future seem especially bright. Whatever her other personal troubles, financial want is not likely to be among them. I doubt she will begrudge this fact in the years to come.

Feminist Sisterhood: Volumes of journals, pamphlets, and responsible treatises call women worldwide to unite in sisterhood and mutual support. This call is a creative response to a public issue: the iron grip of patriarchy on our institutional structures. Many women who have served as surrogate mothers report their extraordinary pleasure at being able to form a bond with a woman who desires but otherwise could not have children, giving her the inestimable gift of a young infant. The potential for building and repeating such bonds in a growing woman-to-woman network of love and affection between genetic mothers, genetrix, and maters, calls for our encouragement when amicable parties are willing and competent to join in this way. Surrogacy is by no means the only or even a central basis for feminist solidarity, but neither is it reprehensible nor deserving of degrading epithets (i.e., mother machines, cows, breeders, baby sellers, etc.).

It is unfortunate that society did not stand ready to help Mary Beth Whitehead and Elizabeth Stern preserve the bonds they began to establish but which shattered in the heat of personal troubles writ large in public courtroom litigation. Our patriarchal society is notoriously intolerant of feminism. The structure of law in this case exacerbates the personal troubles of Mary Beth and Elizabeth, artificially pitting them in adversarial opposition rather than calling forth their mutual interests as multiple parents.

Critics should note that most surrogate reproduction agreements between multiple parents do not land in court, *even in the absence of equity establishing legislation.* Indeed, it is the parties to traditional conjugal nuclear marriages who find themselves in court with considerably greater frequency arguing over the best interests of their children. I suspect that the astoundingly quiet consummation and fulfillment of nearly all other multiple parenting arrangements effected through surrogacy draws deeply on real bonds of sisterhood for success, strength, and meaning. We must be careful not to foil this potential for feminist bonding.

In the case at hand, Melissa will do well to understand that it was unusual for sisterhood to collapse, for her mater to be selected juridically (Judge Sorkow arranged for Elizabeth Stern to sign adoption papers immediately following the reading of his custody decision). Reading his opinion, hopefully Melissa will grant Judge Sorkow now only wisdom but also the latitude for fallibility we all need when making difficult decisions based on necessarily limited data. In the mature resolution of her own personal troubles, Melissa may find the strength, insight, and inclination to mend the broken bonds of sisterhood between her genetic mother/genetrix and her mater. Melissa did not cause these bonds to break and it is not her responsibility to call forth conciliation, but we can give her every support if she should be so spunky as to try. If she does, she should realize, however, that a long history of patriarchal patterns is stacked against her.

Inter-Class Solidarity: The potential for feminist bonding parallels a novel opening for solidarity between economist classes based on shared interests in children. Critics have correctly noted that present surrogacy arrangements are asymmetrical: the surrogate mother is almost invariably of lower class standing than the genetic father. None that I know of however, have argued for mechanisms that could restore the balance somewhat, such as charitable foundations who could fund surrogacy reproduction when the participants involved could not afford it. Indeed, a portion of the fees now going to attorneys could be legislatively diverted to capitalize this proposed foundation.

Short of such funding, however, other opportunities for improved inter-class relations based on surrogate reproduction and multiple parenting should not be ignored. For example, the Sterns agreed to provide Mary Beth Whitehead with "an annual picture and letter report of progress" detailing Melissa's development (Sorkow, 1987:31). This minimal communication is more significant and interpersonally meaningful than generally occurs between most upper middle-class and working-class families.

Giddens (1981) convincingly shows that class relations in industrialized societies are far more complexly textured than orthodox marxists (or most of the more conservative sociologists, for that matter) are willing to grant. Recognizing and acting on class complexity is a public issue which to date has received little if any legislative consideration. We now have an opportunity for action. The many-faceted matrix of class/parent relationships *theoretically possible* in multiple parenthood echoes Gidden's account of class as a variegated social phenomenon. Surrogate reproduction agreements, however, *move concretely*, enacting these possibilities in reality, giving birth to a new form of complex inter-class relation based in multiple parenthood roles. This new inter-class relation provides a structure — and well-being of multiple-parented children provides motivation -- for calling forth deep mutual understanding across class lines. This opportunity, as a public issue, should not be lightly rejected.

Ethnic Heritage and Communal Legacies: Melissa also carries forward, through her genetic makeup and socialization by her pater, William Stern, a very special legacy that rises from the ashes of World War II. In examining the actual features of Melissa's biography, it is sobering to realize that shortly after Elizabeth Stern learned in late 1979 that she had multiple sclerosis and should avoid pregnancy, William Stern became the last surviving member of all branches of his family to escape the Nazi Holocaust when his mother died in 1983 (Brail, 1987; Sorkow, 1987). While some critics condemn the presumed egocentric biological snobbery of men who use extraordinary means to become genetic fathers, such condemnation is wholly unpardonable and insensitive in this case. It is hard to underestimate or feel unsympathetic to the significance William Stern was entitled to place on becoming a genetic father given the intersection of his personal biography with the public issue of genocide. Melissa's inheritance is not simply genetic, it is communal, religious, historic. She has received a special legacy to treasure. To infer otherwise, even remotely, commits a most reprehensible act of anti-semitism and is an immense disservice to William Stern. We should turn with welcome to the emancipatory possibilities created by surrogacy for preserving ethnic and communal identities threatened with extinction.

Orphans Reconsidered: Finally, critics have argued vehemently that surrogacy is a slap in the face to orphaned children who have not been, and may never be adopted. Mellown (1985) makes this case more cogently than most. The essence of the argument is that surrogacy should not be permitted unless adoptable children are first placed in loving and supportive homes. There are several problems with this reasoning, although Mellown's sympathies are clearly admirable. First, an assumption is made that life in orphanages or with foster parents is necessarily injurious and unsatisfactory. In fact, many such settings are far safer and more nurturant than many so-called "normal" homes which continue to spawn nightmarish public records of child neglect, abuse, and injury. Second, many institutionalized children have serious problems requiring the specialized attention of a trained, resident staff. Third, while the adoption drought may not be quite so serious as Judge Sorkow (1987) painted it, it is still severe. Fourth, critics should note that adoption procedures are also class biased in invidious ways. Members of the middle class much more easily demonstrate the characteristics deemed appropriate during screening by adoption agency personnel. Finally, if there is a major group of competent, healthy children who really need homes (an unanalyzed and untested assumption at this point), this is a public issue *in its own right*. It is not solved by banning surrogacy. Childless couples should not be held anymore responsible than anyone else for providing homes for children who lack adequate maters and paters. Childless persons should be asked to do no more than to share equitably in a scheme that distributes adoptable children to maters and paters across the board.

An unnecessary private trouble is thrust on Melissa by writers who conflate the issues of surrogacy and adoption. Melissa must not be given any reason to think that she might be "taking someone else's place" anymore than is the proverbial kid next door. Nor should youngsters with institutionalized, non-familial maters and paters be encouraged to think their lives diminished or degraded by the fact of Melissa's or anyone else's existence. At the same time, if surrogacy serves as a catalyst for rethinking our adoption/orphanage situation and related public policies, so much the better. This, too, is a positive and potentially emancipatory outcome.

Conclusion: Space for Melissa Stern

Scurrilous commentators wrongly impugn not only the motives of the Whiteheads and the Sterns, but also denigrate the morality, sanity, and civic responsibility of any person who dares enter a surrogate reproduction agreement (for especially vituperative examples, see Corea, 1985: 213-249; and Pollitt, 1987). I believe the language and derogatory labeling used in these pseudo-rational accounts is harmful, not only to multiple parents and children generally, but in this specific case to the Whiteheads, the Sterns, and especially to Melissa. Elsewhere, I call attacks of this type a form of "intellectual violence" which hurts rather than emancipates (Hill, 1985). We must be more careful to comment on public issues in ways that separate public concerns from private troubles. We do well to keep in mind that real people will read privately what we write in public.

Charges of criminal baby selling, class exploitation, sexism, unconscionable selfishness, and biological bigotry have issued from journalists (some even claiming — falsely — to be feminist) who write about surrogate parenting. If such charges were true and tied intrinsically to surrogate reproduction *per se* in especially destructive ways, then it might be justified to heap injury, reproach, and opprobrium upon private people who want nothing more radical than to have babies and rear families. Considered reflection suggests, however, that these charges are not true, nor are they problems unique or intrinsic to surrogate reproduction. Persons interested seriously in Melissa Stern's legal and social history are well advised to read the full text of Judge Sorkow's (1987) decision. In it, one finds the surrogacy is not the focal point of the case. Rather, it is Melissa Stern, her needs, her dependencies, her future. Baby "M" is not a symbol for abstracted social causes, it is a pseudonym of an actual person who will laugh, play, cry, and grow to maturity in our communal midst. As fellow humans, it is our job to support her as we can. As a sociologist, I have tried to explain for her that she is not a freak and that her parents are not ogres, that neither she nor her parents are in any way responsible for the storm of controversy, charges and counter charges that greeted her birth. As with any life, Melissa's is worth celebrating and protecting. I am moved by Judge Sorkow's (1987: 121) closing comment:

> *Melissa needs stability and peace, so that she can be nurtured in a loving environment free from chaos and sheltered from the public eye.*

I really do not know why persons want to become parents, it seems such a lot of work, worry, and — often as not — disappointment and heartache. On the other hand, neither do I know why some among us are so bent on viciously punishing those who would move mountains to become parents. I suspect a long, repressive, right-wing hidden agenda motivates these intolerant hacks, but an explication of my suspicions would take us well beyond the scope of this chapter. What I do know is that we must all apparently remind ourselves that we are talking about real parents, real babies, and real futures. We could do much worse than heed Judge Sorkow's closing admonition.

The facts attending Melissa Stern's arrival in the human community instructively demonstrate the unfolding of personal biography in the context of social institutions, the weaving of distinctive tapestries with private woof and public warp. The sociological imagination expands our ability to understand and comprehend these interlacing patterns, to rescue family and parenthood from myopic, hypocritical conflation, to explore the vitality and variety of human invention. Human society is not fixed, but experimental, malleable by self-determined citizens working with mutual understanding to reach widespread social cooperation. Melissa Stern has already given us a great gift, an opportunity to celebrate her life by seeking emancipatory futures for us all. In return, we can give Melissa the gift of privacy, peace, and freedom — a space of her own.

Acknowledgement

The insightful and helpful comments made by Professor Mary Jo Deegan on an earlier version of this chapter are gratefully acknowledged.

References

Barrett, Michele, and Mary McIntosh (1982), *The Anti-Social Family*. London: Verso Editions.

Bernard, Jessie (1972/1982), *The Future of Marriage*. New Haven: Yale University Press.

Brail, Herbert (1987), Public lecture on surrogate motherhood, Albion College, April 28.

Corea, Gena (1985), *The Mother Machine: Reproductive Technologies from Artificial Insemination to Artificial Wombs.* New York: Harper and Row.

Deegan, Mary Jo, and Michael R. Hill (1987), *Women and Symbolic Interaction.* Boston: Allen and Unwin.

Giddens, Anthony (1981), *The Class Structure of Advanced Societies.* Revised edition. New York: Harper and Row.

--------. (1987a), *Social Theory and Modern Sociology.* Stanford: Stanford University Press.

--------. (1987b), *Sociology: A Brief but Critical Introduction.* 2nd edition. San Diego: Harcourt Brace Jovanovich.

Goffman, Erving (1974/1986), *Frame Analysis: An Essay on the Organization of Experience.* Boston: Northeastern University Press.

Hanley, Robert (1987a), "Father of Baby M Granted Custody; Contract Upheld," *New York Times*, April 1, pp. 1 and 12.

--------. (1987b), "Seven-Week Trial Touched Many Basic Emotions," *New York Times*, April 1, p. 13.

Harvard Law Review (1986), "Rumpelstiltskin Revisited: The Inalienable Rights of Surrogate Mothers," Vol. 99, No. 8 (June), pp. 1936-1955.

Hill, Michael R. (1984), "Epistemology, Axiology, and Ideology in Sociology," *Mid-American Review of Sociology*, Vol. 9, No. 2, pp. 59-77.

--------. (1985), "Intellectual Violence, Democratic Legitimation and the War Over the Family," *Midwest Feminist Papers*, Vol. 5, pp. 13-19.

Hollinger, Joan Heifetz (1985), "From Coitus to Commerce: Legal and Social Consequences of Noncoital Reproduction." *University of Michigan Journal of Law Reform*, Vol., 18, No. 4 (Summer), pp. 865-932.

Katz, Avi (1986), "Surrogate Motherhood and the Baby-Selling Laws," *Columbia Journal of Law and Social Problems*, Vol. 20, No. 1, pp. 1-53.

Kristeva, Julia   (1974/1986), *About Chinese Women*. Translated by Anita Barrows. New York: Marion Boyars.

Mead, George Herbert   (1934), *Mind, Self and Society: From the Standpoint of a Social Behaviorist*. Chicago: University of Chicago Press.

Mellown, Mary Ruth   1985, "An Incomplete Picture: The Debate about Surrogate Motherhood," *Harvard Women's Law Journal*, Vol. 8, Spring, pp. 231-246.

Mills, C. Wright   (1959), *The Sociological Imagination*. London: Oxford University Press.

New York Times   (1987), "Excerpts from the Ruling on Baby M," April 1, p. 13.

Pollitt, Katha   (1987), "The Strange Case of Baby M," *The Nation*, Vol. 244, No. 20 (May 23), pp. 667, 682-686, and 688.

Poster, Mark   (1978), *Critical Theory of the Family*. New York: Seabury Press.

Reinharz, Shulamit   (1979/1984), *On Becoming a Social Scientist: From Survey Research and Participant Observation to Experiential Analysis*. New Brunswick: Transaction Books.

Rubin, Lillian Breslow   (1979), *Worlds of Pain: Life in the Working Class Family*. New York: Basic Books.

Schutz, Alfred (1971), *Collected Papers*. 3 Vols. 3rd unchanged edition. The Hague: Martinus Nijhoff.

Scott, Hilda   (1984), *Working Your Way to the Bottom: The Feminization of Poverty*. London: Pandora Press.

Shipp, E.R.   (1987), "Larger Issues of Surrogacy," *New York Times*, April 1, pp. 1 and 13.

Sorkow, Harvey R.   (1987), Opinion, In the Matter of Baby "M", a pseudonym for an actual person, Superior Court of New Jersey, Chancery Division, Family Part, Bergen County, Docket No. FM-25314-86E, issued March 31, 1987. Mimeo. 121 pages.

Taft, Jessie (1915/1987), "The Women Movement and Social Consciousness," reprinted in M.J. Deegan and M.R. Hill, eds.,

Women and Symbolic Interaction. Boston: Allen and Unwin, 1987, pp. 19-50.

The Gift Mother

*A Proposed Ritual for
the Integration of Surrogacy into Society*

MARY JO DEEGAN

The Baby M Case -- as it is popularly called (e.g. Fleming 1987) --is a human tragedy. Two families and their joint child are caught in the vicious web of American corporate life. They are betwixt and between sexism, capitalism, bureaucracy, the court system, the medical establishment, lawyers, the mass media, and family hysteria (Turner, 1969, Young, 1976a and b; Young and Massey, 1978; Deegan, 1987). As one journalist melodramatically describes it: "it's a tale of sex and money, love and greed, eager hope and cruel betrayal. It's the stuff of soap operas, cheap tabloids, and pulp fiction (Gallagher, p. 27)." It is much more than this, of course, but it is being writ large in the popular media in these terms and this public response is part of the tragedy.

In this chapter I advance a few simple ideas:

First, the situation of the baby and families is tragic.

Second, this situation emerges from the structure of American life.

Third, this situation of surrogate mothering could be one of celebration.

Fourth, surrogate mothering involves a rite of passage unsupported by anti-structural or liminal rules and symbols.

Fifth, the failure to celebrate the community drama of surrogate mothering has left a vacuum of meaning that is being filled by stigma and "bad faith."

And sixth, learning from the Baby M fiasco, and thereby reincorporating and reinterpreting the families' pain as a gift to the community, can help us generate a ritual of love, cooperation, and giving.

I.   The Tragedy: The Narrative

A tragedy is a social drama, in this case a lived one (Turner, 1969, Goffman, 1959) with disastrous results. The structure of the narrative contains fatal flaws leading to the unhappy ending. In my recounting of the drama, I include the problematic interactions, institutions, and roles as structural, not interpersonal, elements generating this American tragedy. A published summary of the case is used here to present the narrative, because it is succinct and shows a media construction of the event including popular typifications of institutional roles. (Thomas and Znaniecki, 1918-1920; Reinharz, 1987)

> *For $10,000*, Mary Beth Whitehead agreed to bear a child and give her to Bill Stern and his wife. After *Baby M* was born, Mary Beth *changed her mind. She refused the ten grand* and kept *Baby M* for four months, fleeing to Florida after a *New Jersey court* granted the Sterns *temporary custody.* (Gallagher, 1987: 27. Italics added here are to be discussed in a later segment of this chapter.)
>
> The baby is kidnapped by the surrogate mother and hides from the police for four months. The ten-year-old half-sister of Baby M hears a *strange man's voice,* and runs out into the hall to see what's happening. Three men stand in front of her sister's room. They see the crib. *One man snatches up the baby and runs toward the front door. Maybe it looks like a kidnapping, but it's all perfectly kosher: the Men are officers of the law.* (Gallagher, 1987: 27. Italics added here and to be discussed in a later segment of this chapter.)

The Sterns ultimately regain custody after extensive litigation that is accompanied by sensationalized press coverage. Both parents and their respective spouses want the child. Their lives are disrupted by two antagonistic definitions of parental rights. They are embedded in a legal snare that is costly, lengthy, public, and adversarial. Lawyers, judges, courtroom personnel, the police and clerks are involved in making a public decision on which parent has the greater right to raise the child. Other paid "experts" include psychologists and medical personnel, first as "service providers" and later as "witnesses" in the courtroom. These parents and their families are not united by relationships and obligations of love and duty. They are tied by contract law and as "patients" in an adversarial system mediated by paid experts, often from the middle and upper middle class. These meanings and relationships are emerging from a capitalistic society organized by bureaucratic rules and controlled by men (Deegan, 1987). In this society, birth is medicalized by a patriarchal bureaucracy instead of celebrated by the family and community (Ehrenreich and English, 1978; Corea, 1977; Ruzek discusses the variety of feminist options in 1979). Medical settings, moreover, are particularly inhospitable environments for times of celebration, grief, or community renewal (Deegan, forthcoming).

II.   The Possibility of Celebrating Surrogate Mothering and Liminality

Surrogate mothering has the potential to be a life-giving, community-renewing ritual: a gift of life (Titmuss, 1971). This potential has been enacted for many people -- approximately 600 to date (Quindlen, 1987: 25) -- and we need information about their lives and responses. We also need to generate community dramas and rituals as part of our process of being human, living and dying. The first need, for a research agenda, is beyond the scope or intent of this chapter. The second need, a community defined process of celebration, is addressed here.

Surrogate mothering can be a positive, multivocal symbol (Turner, 1969) pointing to the previous barrenness and the promised fertility. The expansion of family through new others, both within and outside the family, shows the flexibility of love and community. The baby born of a surrogate mother is both of the flesh -- a member by blood -- and of the law, a member by contract and law (Schneider, 1969). Surrogate mothering is a gift from one family to another. It is a gift relationship, (Mauss, 1966) not "baby selling" on a shameful market. (See Cheal, 1987, on the problems of gift exchanges in capitalist societies.)

In order to suggest a community direction, I offer here a model of celebration for this gift relationship. In light of my assumptions, I will call a "surrogate mother" a "gift mother." Several stages of ritual action are delineated, and each stage has a set of appropriate symbols, actions, and relationships. Clearly this is a skeletal idea to offer for community decision-making.

The Rite of Passage

In 1906, Arnold Van Gennepp (1966) articulated for Western society the rich and varied world of rituals in nonmodern societies. His work has been elaborated by Victor Turner in a series of books (e.g., 1967, 1969, 1974, 1982). Both theorists examine rites of passage as processual, with ceremonies of *seperation, marginality (or liminality),* and *reaggregation.* The beginning and ending of status changes mark the boundaries between the time of transition. The marginal point, betwixt and between statuses, is often emotionally charged, symbolically powerful, and organized according to rules different from everyday ones. This liminal period is "anti-structural" in the sense of difference not opposition (Turner, 1969). Turner and Van Gennepp's ideas organize my ideas for surrogate mothering as a celebration of a birth and its gift of love from one family to another.

Rites of Separation

Stage 1: The Search for a Gift Mother and Family

The decision to search for a gift mother begins the ritual. A process different from "everyday" family procreation occurs. It can start within the home, with family and friends; or in bureaucratic settings, with doctors, social workers, and lawyers. This ritual, however it begins, should be controlled by the family initiating the search and their circle of intimates. "Experts" are needed in the form of midwives, community responsive lawyers, and auxilliary medical institutions. They consult and advise the new family-to-be. The process of having a baby and searching for a mother are not "expert services" in the hands of professionals, but community and family processes.

Stage 2: Agreeing to Begin the Pregnancy

The main participants in surrogate mothering are:
1) the father and his intimate partner
2) the mother and her intimate partner(s) and children
3) the midwife
4) the contract brokers, probably lawyers

Each member of this process needs to meet face-to-face, discuss their options fully and examine possible scenarios, both positive and negative in their outcomes. Ritual food should be shared on these occasions, following other ritual menus served at times of celebration in our culture. Coffee and cakes, for example, are both modest yet meaningful foods. The possibility of meeting on more than one occasion in order to reach an agreement needs to be stressed. The voluntary nature of the exchange, the need for cooperation and openness should be key themes. This can be structured into the discussion in a series of ways. Failure to reach an agreement can be incorporated into the ritual at this point.

Rites of Liminality

Stage 3: Insemination

Insemination should occur in comfortable surroundings; this is a home/community/family event. Comfort, food, and talk should surround it. The emphasis on the naturalness of giving birth is integral to the process. At this stage, all of the participants are "liminal"; betwixt and between family and birth. The process of insemination should be defined as pleasurable, an enactment of a deep bond and commitment as well as a biological event. The act of insemination is not complex, nor it require expensive equipment. One account frequently repeated in the press is the use of turkey baster for the transfer of semen (e.g., I heard this story at a presentation by a lawyer in the firm that contracted "Baby M", Herbert Brail, 28 April, 1987; See also Fleming, 1987: 27). This is a good example of how easy the process is to complete as well as a kind of "nonsacred," problematic way to approach this act. The possibility of a child comparing his or her birth to the process of baking a dead bird is real and symbolically devastating. The incongruity of the instrument to the task partially explains why it is repeated as an anecdote, but it is also symbolically barren for a human act of great magnitude. "Professionals" conduct artificial inseminations in clinics and "doctors charge as much as $500 per insemination" (Gallagher, 1987: 27). This drama is similarly problematic, symbolizing class, gender, and knowledge differences based on inequality.

Artificial insemination can be done in the home, in a more relaxed and celebratory atmosphere. This gives more control to the participants instead of "experts." This also avoids the scandalous outcome of another surrogate case where the gift mother and father decided at the last minute to avoid the clinic and engage in intercourse in a nearby hotel. The father left his wife to join the gift mother and her husband, or so the sensational account states, leaving the wife both abandoned and without a child (Lavoie, 1987). This surrogate tragedy emerged from an attempt to have the participants control the process, avoid the dehumanizing space and actions in medical settings, and the intrinsic voyerism of professionals controlling a family event. (I refer to voyerism in its symbolic, Freudian, dimension and not as an accusation against practioners. For a discussion of my dramaturgical use of Freudian thought see Deegan, 1987, 1986, 1983.))

Stage 4: Pregnancy

Prenatal care is important and guided by the midwife. Small gift exchanges, tokens of concern such as cards and flowers, would be appropriate. Concern for mother and baby are of paramount importance: they are the central figures in the drama at this point. The woman takes on the role of the pregnant mother (Mead, 1934) in "everyday" pregnancy, but in surrogacy the entire family is symbolically included at this stage. Acknowledging that they are all giving a gift and sharing their lives through the gift mother honors their contributions. The importance of including everyone at this point is vital. Thus, one gift mother distressingly testified at a legislative hearing that her

children listened to the baby's heartbeat through a stethoscope
and felt him move.

"I didn't know they were falling in love with their brother," she
said, sobbing. (Firestone, 1987: 4B)

Acknowledging the family's gift to another family would give these
children, and other children, the meaningful recognition and honor
they deserve.

The father and his wife can follow the model of "involved father"
already existing in our culture. They are "expecting" a baby. Reinharz
(1987) poignantly discusses how "expecting a baby" becomes a role
integral to the self during pregnancy. The gift mother is "expecting a
surrogate baby", her family is "expecting a surrogate baby
sibling/child", and the father and the adopted mother are "expecting
their baby" and are "parents-to-be."

As the end of the pregnancy nears, every effort to insure the comfort
and concerns of the mother and her family must be made. A ritual
questioning ceremony would provide a stage for reaffirming
commitments, assuring that the participants know that doubts and
renewal are incorported in the process. Every effort to avoid an
adversarial ritual must be made. Therefore, the parents-to-be should
avoid using legal pressure and language arising from contract law.
This ritual must assume good will in a gift relationship. The gift
mother and her family must be supported in their responses and
generosity. Any of their questions would be seriously considered and
answered. Their concerns at this point are part of their gift.

Stage 5: Delivery

The delivery ritual builds on the present midwifery model (See
Ruzek, 1979). A close relationship between the gift mother-to-be and
the midwife is developed during the pregnancy. The working
relationship for these partners is emphasized. The woman delivers the
baby, the midwife assists her in this process. (The medicalized,
bureaucractic language states that doctors deliver babies!) The
cooperative model developed for mothers and midwives can be
adapted for other services employed during the gift delivery as well.

The two families should share this time of anticipation again following the "involved father" model. The mother and child would preferably be "at home" or minimally in a "birthing center."

Rites of Reaggregation

Stage 6: Completing the Families' Transitions

When the gift mother delivers the baby, the transition from the gift family to the new family occurs. Again, a brief ceremony of giving, gratitude, thanks, and celebration marks this transition. Assuring the gift mother's children that they are part of this process, demystifies the birth and exchange. It connects their emotions, actions, and relationships to generous new parents. Bonding does not occur only in newborns, it is part of continuing life.

The very language of "the Baby M case" reveals its divisive nature. The child has two names, Sara and Melissa, so an anonymous letter "M" is arbitarily used. The struggle is "a case" -- a legal battle with antagonists. The desperate mother kidnapped the baby, violating any trust between her and the new family. The anguish they felt about the possible injury or death to the baby is awful and frightening. The entry of the uniformed state, the violence of the taking and return, point to another deep cultural violation (Geertz, 1973). In the Baby M case, the gift mother was increasingly concerned, worried, and coerced. Failure to respond to her valid worries at this stage may have precipitated the later pain. It certainly allowed her doubts to grow and deepen. Perhaps attention to her fears would have resulted in the end of the surrogate mothering, but certainly the terrible tragedy following the birth would have been prevented.

III. Surrogate Mothering and the Social Construction of Stigma

Baby M symbolically stands for the deep conflicts in this society over surrogate mothering. I would like to briefly address these more general issues here. There is a widespread media attack labeling surrogate mothering in a pernicious manner. In other words, at this historical moment we are witnessing the social construction of a stigma: surrogate mothering is being labeled as a discrediting attribute. (Goffman, 1961; Becker, 1963). This labeling is occurring in both the "legitimate" and more sensational printed media.

In Table 1, I compiled a series of discrediting terms and statements found in popular magazines published in 1987 on the Baby M situation. (Italicized passages in the narrative cited on pg. 92 here show both the use of denigrating language and the stressful reality of anonymous agents who act for the court system.)

TABLE 1. STIGMA CONSTRUCTION FROM THE POPULAR PRESS

AUTHOR	PHRASE OR STATEMENT
Gallagher	A great soap opera; surrogate mothers are really surrogate wives (p. 27)
	a kind of Frankenstein's monster, a moral horror brought on by science-out-of-control (. 27)
	The advant-garde of this destructive force is the surrogate mother herself (p.29)
	Like prostitution, surrogate mothering makes one of the most intimate acts a commercial, and therefore impersonal, transation. Like indentured servitude, it permits an individual to sell away her personal autonomy (p.30, boldface)
Fleming	an act that felt a little too much like conceptual adultery (p. 37)
	that M stands for -- Motherhood (p. 37)
	Impersonal procreation and impersonal destruction --do they go hand in hand? (p. 37)
	Surrogacy for me, I have finally concluded, would not be a moral choice (p. 87)
Firestone	"Ban sale of babies, surrogate mom begs lawmakers" (Headline, B Section, *Detroit News*)
	The bill's sponsor...said surrogate contracts exploit women and make babies "an object to be bought and sold like new furniture for the living room or a new car." (p. 1B)

(Legal advisor's testimony of imagined future pyschological damage) "My real mommy never wanted me. All she wanted was the money for which she sold me." (p. 4B, last statement in the article.)

Although not all language is stigmatizing, the non-discrediting view is usually framed as the "other side" and the authors of these articles claim they oppose surrogate mothering. Popular radio and television reports echo this printed response. The exchange of money appears particularly problematic, but the gift mother is engaged in an extreme act of generosity. Is she to be unthanked? Unrewarded? Frequently, money in a capitalist society transforms human actions into commodities. Workers clearly sell their labor and lose control over their lives in the process, but is this voluntary gift exchange the same process? I think not. To give money as a token of appreciation, honor, and good intent needs to be stated ritually. There is no price for a human child. The father is not buying a slave, or "a new piece of furniture" as one opponent states. The father is honoring another woman who has borne him a child. The father of the child is not buying his own child. The overwhelming majority of gift mothers have understood this. Their families have understood this, and their compassion is being redefined by a variety of professional labelers.

The mass media, in particular, have actively stigmatized surrogate mothering. They are, to use Becker's term, "moral entrepreneurs" who profit from the labeling of deviant behavior. Gallagher, a particularly virulent opponent, denigrates surrogate mothers' generosity and good faith by writing that: "They cheerfully produce infants and hand them over, without admitting pain or grief or guilt (p. 29)." She labels the surrogate mothers as suffering from "temporary insanity" (p. 30), a gross distortion of these mothers' views of the world. All the articles that I found between April and May of 1987 were written by women, moreover, making it appear as if this is a special "woman's topic" in the press's division of labor. (Feminist authors in the scholarly presses are not motivated by money, and they raise important questions of race and class biases. Banning the surrogate process is not a way to resolve these problems, however.)

Surrogate mothering is often treated as identical with a variety of ways to obtain a baby that are different from the two parents/married/birth couple. Thus, adoption, in vitro fertilization, artificial insemination, and surrogacy are often compared simultaneously. The front cover of *Life* printed in large type: "The Try-Everything World of *Baby Craving*." (Quindlen, 1987) thereby combining very different technologies and behaviors into one group. Duelli Klein documents atrocious inequalities and injustices condoned by "experts" in reproductive technology, and she discusses them in conjunction with surrogate mothering (1987). She labels all these procedures "disastrous" (p. 92). Similarly, the recent statement by the Roman Catholic leaders forbade "in vitro fertilization, the freezing of embryos and surrogate motherhood, as well as the collection of sperm through masturbation, a necessary corollary of many of the technological methods, including artificial insemination." (Quindlen, 1987: 26).

Because of the widespread alienation and exploitation characterizing capitalist and patriarchal societies, many legitimate fears and problems are emerging from surrogate mothering. Baby M is a symbolic tragedy pointing to our failure to understand and celebrate human life. The first gift mother testified in Michigan that seven years after giving birth to a gift child her family has been destroyed by it:

"It's like looking at the aftermath of a tornado, said the Illinois woman, *under the alias Elizabeth Kane* to protect her identity. "There's so much damage that we don't know where to go for help, where to go to pick up the pieces." (Firestone, 1 B. Italicized phrase points to stigma this gift mother feels.)

As a community we must hear these pleas for respect and recognition. We need a consensus of affirmation and celebration. Stigmatizing these families and their children as buyers and sellers of flesh reveals bad faith on the part of those who label. The comments in Table 1 show the punishing language emerging from the present situation. A celebratory *rite de passage* provides the context of good will needed to forstall this pernicious view of bad faith.

Conclusion

The Baby M case is a rite of passage illuminating the snarl of American life. Its tragic proportions point to the failure of our communities to celebrate life, the horizons of new knowledge, and the posibility of generating a rich world of meaning and symbol based on our experiences and heritage. In our antagonistic world of capitalism, paid experts, bureaucracy, and patriarchy, a time of enrichment has been turned into a world of suspicion and bad faith. I have offered a possible scenario of celebration, based on our tradition of families and birth, midwives, sacraments, and justice. I have borrowed from the traditional worlds of nonmodern people who are not adrift on a sea of anomie. My suggested rite of passage for gift relationships between surrogate familites and parents-to-be also emerges from our modern life with its knowledge of reproduction, anthropology, sociology, and biology. We can enrich and expand life -- if these new powers are in the hands of a democratic people.

Acknowledgement

The staff and participants in the Women, Health and Healing Institute of 1985 and 1986, sponsored by the University of California-San Francisco, School of Nursing, helped me renew my feminist vision in health care services. Special thanks to Virginia Olesen, Sheryl Ruzek, and Adele Clark. The final form of this chapter is, of course, my responsibility.

Bibliography

Becker, Howard S.   1963. *The Outsiders*. New York: Free Press.

Braile, Herbert.   1987. Panel presentation on "Baby M" at Albion College, Albion, MI, 28 April.

Cheal, David   1987. "Showing Them You Love Them: Gift Giving and the Dialectic of Intimacy." *Sociological Review* 35 (Feb.): 150-69.

Corea, Gena. 1977. *The Hidden Malpractice*. New York: Jove/Harcourt, Brace, Javanovich.

Deegan, Mary Jo. Forthcoming. "Holidays as Multiple Realities: Experiencing Good Times and Bad Times after a Disabling Injury." *Journal of Sociology and Social Welfare*.

------. 1987. "American Drama and Ritual." Unpublished book manuscript.

------. 1986. "Sexism in Space: The Freudian Formula in *Star Trek*." In *Eros in the Mind's Eye*, ed. by Donald Palumbo. Westport, CT: Greenwood Press. pp. 209-24.

------. 1983. "A Feminist Frame Analysis of *Star Trek*: Or Feminists Boldly Go Where No Man Has Gone Before." In *Contributions to the Sociology of Art*, ed. by Elit Nikolov. Pp. 486-504.

------. 1978. "The Social Dramas of Erving Goffnma and Victor Turner." *Humanity and Society* 2 (Fall): (February): 33-46.

------ and Michael Stein. 1978. "American Drama and Ritual: Nebraska Football." *International Review of Sport Sociology* 13 (December): 31-44.

------. 1977. "Pornography as a Strip and a Frame." *Sociological Symposium* 20 (Fall): 27-44.

Ehrenreich, Barbara and Deidree English. 1978. *For Her Own Good*. New York: Anchor Press.

Firestone, Joanna. 1987. "Ban Sale of Babies, Surrogate Mom Begs Lawmakers." *The Detroit News* (13 May): 1B, 4B.

Fleming, Anne Taylor. 1987. "Our Fascination with Baby M." *The New York Times Magazine* (29 March): 32-38+.

Gallagher, Maggie. 1987. "Womb to Let." 39 (24 April): 27-30.

Geertz, Clifford. 1973 *Interpretation of Cultures*. New York: Basic Books.

Goffman, Erving. 1974. *Frame Analysis: An Essay on the Organization of Experience*. New York: Harper and Row.

------. 1967. *Interaction Ritual: Essays on Face-to-Face Behavior*. New York: Anchor Books.

------. 1963. *Stigma: Notes on the Management of Spoiled Identity.* Englewood Cliffs, NJ: Prentice-Hall.

------. 1961. *Asylums: Essays on the Social Situation of Mental Patients and Other Inmates.* Garden City, NY: Doubleday.

------. 1959. *The Presentation of Self in Everyday Life.* New York: Doubleday.

Klein, Renate Duelli. 1984. "Taking the Egg from the One and the Uterus from the Other." *Development: Seeds of Change* 4: 92-97.

Lavoie, Claire. 1987. "Husband Runs Off With Surrogate Mom!" *Weekly World News* (26 May): 39.

Mauss, Marcel. 1966. *The Gift.* Tr. Ian Cunnison, Intro. by E. E. Evans Pritchard. London: Cohen and West.

Mead, George H. 1934. *Mind. Self and Society: From the Standpoint of a Social Behaviorist,* ed. by Charles W. Morris. Chicago: University of Chicago Press.

Nebraska Feminist Sociology Collective, eds. 1987. *Feminist Ethics and Social Science Research.* Lewiston, NY: The Edwin Mellen Press.

Reinharz, Shula. 1987. In *Women and Symbolic Interaction,* ed. by Mary Jo Deegan and Michael R. Hill. Waltham, MA: Allen & Unwin. Pp. 229-50.

Ruzek, Sheryl Burt. 1979. *The Women's Health Movement.* New York: Praeger.

Schneider, David. 1969. *American Kinship.* Englewood Cliffs, NJ: Prentice-Hall.

Thomas, W. I. and Florian Znaniecki. 1918-1920. *The Polish Peasant in Europe and America.* Boston: Badger Press.

Titmuss, Richard M. 1971. *The Gift Relationship.* NY: Pantheon Books.

Turner, Victor R. 1974. *Dramas, Fields, and Metaphors: Symbolic Action in Human Society.* Ithaca: Cornell University Press.

------. 1969. *The Ritual Process.* Chicago: Aldine.

------. 1968. *The Drums of Affliction*. Oxford: Clarendon.

------. 1967. *The Forest of Symbols*. Ithaca: Cornell University Press.

Van Gennepp, Arnold. 1966. (c. 1906). *The Rites of Passage*. Chicago: University of Chicago Press.

Young, T.R. 1982. "The Structure of Democratic Communications." Red Feather Institute.

------. 1976a. "Critical Dimensions in Dramaturgical Analysis: Part 1. Red Feather Institute.

------. 1976b. "Critical Dimensions in Dramaturgical Analysis: Part 2. Red Feather Institute.

------ and Garth Massey. 1978. "The Dramaturgical Society." Qualitative Sociology 1 (September): 78: 98.

Sorting Out Motivations
Personal Integrity as the
First Criterion of Moral Action

MICHAEL D. RYAN

Because the very terms of the issue (such as "surrogate motherhood") have become controversial, I am using the term "surrogate pregnancy." In theological perspective what we are talking about is the gift of life and the human role in being custodians of that gift. On this basis, it seems to me that there are some hard questions that must be put to all of the parties involved in a contract for surrogate pregnancy.

As a theologian who stands in the Unitarian-Universalist tradition of the Judeo-Christian heritage, I am not prepared to give a dogmatic "Yes" or "No" to surrogate pregnancy. It is indeed a matter of evaluating the motives and the personal situations of the parties of such an agreement. I was first tempted to reflect on "higher" and "lower" motives on the part of the surrogate female after the manner of Immanuel Kant, the great German philosopher of the Enlightenment. But it seems clear to me that in our society, with its two broad streams of religious and secular thinking, we might categorize the motives as "religious" and "secular" and allow for some preferences, "higher and lower" if you will, within each category.

As for the surrogate in the "Baby M" case, it was reported that the basic religious motive of Mary Beth Whitehead was to give an infertile mother the gift of a child so that God might perhaps give a child to an infertile relative of hers. I think that such bargaining with God is misguided, but I must admit that there is a long religious heritage for such bargaining. But let's assume a sincere desire based on a deep religious conviction that one may in an unusual way participate in bringing the gift of human life to a couple, and so initiate the forming of a family. This could be a possible religious or ethically ideal reason for entering surrogate pregnancy. So there can be different kinds of religious motivations, depending on the kind of religious conviction involved.

Likewise there can be different kinds of secular motivations, depending on the type of ethical convictions involved. A person without any particular beliefs about God, one way or another, might very well determine to give this gift as the noblest thing that one woman might be able to do for another, especially since it would not involve having direct intercourse with the woman's husband. Or, one might do it for the money, and this for a number of reasons that could possibly range from having the cash for a special purpose such as education, improving the lot of the children and family that one already has, having money for a catastrophic illness in the family, or making a down-payment on a home, or refurbishing the house, or buying a new car. So, the reasons for the money could range from the morally serious to the trivial.

But between the religiously and ethically ideal or noble reason of giving a gift and the various reasons that can be purchased with money there is a possible ethical and religious distinction. It has to do with the self-understanding and the personhood of the surrogate woman. If a woman, whether for religious or purely ethical reasons, gives the gift out of the integrity of her own self, as the thing that she wants to do for the couple in question, then the gift is an expression of her own integrity as a person, and as a believer in God, if that is the case.

But if a woman comes to look at surrogate pregnancy simply as a means to an end, then she enters into an instrumental relationship with her own body. If that is the case, then as Dr. Salk, the psychiatrist who testified as an expert witness for the Sterns in the "Baby M" case said, she should think of herself as a "surrogate uterus." Ethically, this is what the great Jewish theologian Martin Buber called "an I-It relation," only she enters into an "I-It relation" not simply with her physical uterus as Dr. Salk thinks, but with the process of pregnancy that involves her whole body for a period of nine months. She is renting her whole body. If it is done strictly for the money, and what it can buy, then it might be considered as a higher type of prostitution on the analogy of renting the use of a physical function of the female body.

I am not suggesting that surrogate pregnancy is always merely instrumental, nor am I denying the right of a woman to enter into that type of contract. In a very real sense all of us who work for a paycheck place our bodies, their energy and capacities, at the disposal of others for specified periods of time. But I am suggesting that anyone contemplating this surrogate role from artificial insemination through carrying the fetus to full term should be sure of her own motives, and of her integrity. She should be honest with her *self* throughout the whole process.

Likewise, the "renting couple" should be sure of her and their own motives and should be prepared to respect the integrity of the surrogate woman throughout the process. What is the moral implication of asking a woman to enter into an "I-It relation" with her uterus? Isn't it asking her to be less than whole during the period of pregnancy? This raises a number of questions as to the nature of a surrogate pregnancy contract and the procedures for entering into it and for carrying out its terms.

Shouldn't there be a provision in the contract for the fetus-bearing female to change her mind? To insist against the will of the woman that she give up the fruit of her womb seems to suggest that she must deny any impulse to a reformulation of the meaning of her integrity that could occur in her moments of contemplation any time during the nine months of pregnancy.

What about the agency that brings parties for surrogate pregnancy together? Shouldn't the parties to such a contract have comparable economic and social status, as well as physical characteristics, so that a court would not always have to find in favor of the renting couple in case of a dispute arising from a change of heart?

Should not the surrogate female agree in advance to intensive pre-conception testing and counseling?

Should not the surrogate female *and* and the renting couple agree to therapy during the period of pregnancy, and be very specific in the contract about the goal of such therapy? This is definitely a moral issue, because, on the one hand, one could move to two ends:

(a) recognize the right of the surrogate mother to change her mind, and so therapy would be conducted from the standpoint of helping her to live out, with integrity, a choice she has made; or,

(b) one could use behaviorist techniques to condition her to the acceptance of the strict terms of her contract, which therapy would include preparation for psychological and well as physical separation from the womb.

Should not post-partem therapy for the surrogate female be paid for by the renting couple, along with all of the therapy involved for the surrogate female?

Such a contract, which allows for the possibility of a change of heart on the part of the surrogate female, and provides a process for that to take place, respects the personhood and the integrity of all persons involved. Without such a provision we have the most unsavory features of the "Baby M" case in which the very real process that Mrs. Whitehead experienced during the pregnancy is denied any serious consideration, so that she is rendered a piece of chattel according to law, and hence her pregnancy a matter of slavery. The consideration of the future welfare and well-being of the child will rightly get primary consideration, but it seems that a significant part of the price for that well-being will have been the forced personal sacrifice of Mrs. Whitehead.

A family formed at the expense of the personal struggle for integrity on the part of the surrogate female is a rather questionable entity. It suggests a "throw away" attitude towards a person that our religious heritage, be it Jewish, Christian or Unitarian-Universalist cannot support. A court and legal system that enforces such a contract against the will of the surrogate mother plays the role of *sicut Deus*, of playing "like God" in the matter. Surely, Mary Beth Whitehead has a claim on the Sterns for any therapy essential for her future well-being as a person and mother.

God is the Creator of Human Life
A Calvinist Defense of Surrogate Parenthood

HERBERT RICHARDSON

The development of technologies which facilitate control over procreation has created a crisis for our understanding of human beings. If we can intend and make babies the same way that we can intend and make automobiles, then babies are products of human labor. They have a cash value; they can be bought and sold; they can be genetically manipulated and destroyed if they are defective. If we describe babies as if they were *things* made by us through the same processes as we make other things, then procreation resembles the activities by which we manufacture products.

The problem with thinking of babies as products is that it undermines the foundations of society because society presupposes that persons are not things (objects), but are subjects possessing intrinsic value and inalienable rights. If human beings are persons and not products, then the activity of procreation must be essentially different from the productive activity by which we make things. Babies are "begotten, not made." Therefore, we can only understand the issues involved in surrogate parenthood if we have an understanding of procreation as essentially different from manufacturing, a productive process.

The Procreation of Persons

At the present time, there is no well-developed philosophy of procreation which stands as an alternative to materialistic accounts. The Marxist can give an account of baby-making which interprets the activity as a form of human labor which produces a value-added commodity. Even so, that same Marxist vigorously defends the rights of every person as a free subject, deserving of justice. Therefore, the

Marxist believes that, in the course of life, a baby acquires the dignity characteristic of a personal subject. But where and how does this occur?

We need, I believe, a positive description of the procreative process which can function as an alternative to the materialistic description of procreation as an activity "manufacturing babies." We need this because we must account for our belief that babies are persons possessing full human dignity and inalienable rights. A baby is never property; at no time at all is s/he lacking rights. S/he is always a subject, never an object. This is why, I presume, Judge Sorkow can focus his custody decision in terms of "what is best for Melissa" rather than what is best for either of her parents, for Melissa possesses no less rights than the two persons who are in conflict over her custody. She is a person, not a property, from the very beginning.

We understand how we produce property; but do we understand how persons come into being. Do we make them? Are they beings we create? Do they drive "rights" and "dignity" from us? Do they have to "earn" our respect? Probably all Americans will agree that "personhood" and "rights" do not derive from society or from parents because this view is stated in our Bill of Rights. We no longer accept the Roman view of father-right whereby the newborn child was laid on the ground and the father could bestow life upon it by picking it up and receiving it or he could condemn it to death by letting it remain on the ground. We believe that babies are persons, possessing the full dignity that every other person has. But how does a baby come to be a rights-possessing person?

Perhaps the most articulate alternative to the Marxist account of procreation as a form of production is the Catholic view. The Catholic view understands sexual intercourse not as the cause of conception, but as a condition in relation to which God can act directly to create a human being. On the Catholic view, the creator of the baby is God and not human activity. Yet, the Catholic account of normative procreation seems to consist primarily in counseling *against human interference* with the processes of "nature." Nature, on the Catholic view, functions as an instrument of God's creative activity; therefore to respect God's activity means not to interfere (i.e., "no contraception," "no *in vitro* fertilization," etc.). Yet to understand the *positive* meaning of these non-interferences, we must have a fuller account of nature's normativity.

The Problem of "Contracts"

There are various theories which attempt to account for the condition of intrinsic dignity and alienable rights of persons: theological, psychological, political. A theological account of rights is enshrined in the founding constitution of America: "we are endowed with inalienable rights by our Creator." A psychological/philosophical alternative explains that persons are (by definition) characterized by a capacity for "freedom" which qualifies them to be subjects. Finally, a political account might simply claim that "rights" are *there*, anterior to society, and cannot be taken away without destroying the social compact.

What is characteristic of every theory of the origin of rights is that it implies that we must *acknowledge* them; we do not *bestow* them. We do not create rights; we do not make persons. Persons originate beyond our powers to create or uncreate. Persons are subjects not objects. We acknowledge them as such.

Because babies are persons, they cannot be treated as property. Babies cannot be bought or sold. To allow persons to be bought or sold—or exterminated when they are useless or not longer desired— would be to allow the policies of Auschwitz to become the public philosophy. Therefore, agreements governing the relations of surrogate parents must be conceived to be different from the kinds of contracts by which we regulate the buying and selling of things. Even to argue that laws governing contracts which regulate buying and selling set a precedent for agreements among surrogate parents is to misconceive the character of the surrogate agreement.

Those who oppose the practice of surrogate parenthood frequently attempt to disqualify the practice by characterizing the surrogate agreement as a "contract to buy and sell babies." Those who defend the practice argue that such agreements are not "contracts to buy and sell," but resemble adoption procedures. In adoption, what is at stake is not the transference of *ownership* of property, but the transference of *custody*, or the responsibility to care for someone under conditions which respect that someone's full personhood and rights. In fact, failure to treat the adopted baby as a person can result in the termination of custody rights. Hence, *adoption procedures* are agreements relating to persons whereas *contracts to buy and sell* are agreements relating to property.

There are many kinds of agreements other than those which regulate the buying and selling of things. The vows of marriage, the adoption of children, and the promises we make to one another are all agreements among persons. Society originates out of a network of such personal agreements which have no other object than the creation of the social order. It is difficult for me to understand why surrogacy agreements should not be understood and formulated as these kinds of promises which are constitutive of all marriage, most adoptions, and society at large. Not to construe them in this way could suggest that babies born from such arrangements *might* be property.

The Exchange of Money

To the extent that we have failed to describe and control the agreements relating to surrogate parenthood in analogy with adoption agreements, there will be confusion about the legitimacy of surrogacy. A similar kind of confusion arises at a second point, namely, the meaning of the exchange of money in conjunction with surrogate arrangements.

The fact that surrogate parenthood involves the "exchange of money" has led some opponents of this practice to charge that it is a form of prostitution where sex is bought and sold as if it were a commercial product. Most defenders of surrogacy do not argue that it is legitimate to buy and sell sexual services (though there are some who do so argue). Rather, they argue that the money exchange should be regarded as other than "payment for services rendered." In this volume, for example, Professor Deegan suggests that the money exchange should be regarded as a "gift of honor and appreciation." Others argue that the money exchange is compensation for lost time rather than for specific services. Generally speaking, both proponents and opponents of surrogate motherhood agree that money should not be exchanged for "services rendered."

Because the way we interpret the money-exchange implies a way of looking at the baby (i.e., product or person?), it is crucially important that the money exchange in surrogacy never be construed as "payment for services." If it is, then the baby can be regarded as a product rather than a person. Therefore, just as we have argued that the *agreement* between the surrogate parents must be construed as a form of "adoption procedure" rather than as a "contract to buy and sell," so we argue that the *money exchange* should be regarded as a gift or as a compensation for time lost, rather than as a payment for labor. Only in this way can we protect the claim that the baby is fully a person and not property. We must maintain a consistency of terminology in describing the practice of surrogacy.

Confusion arises in our society because of the assumption that because some money is exchanged to purchase commodities, all exchange of money must be for this reason. Yet all money exchange is not for the sake of payment or purchase. Money is also used among humans as a gift; and the function of gifts is to establish and to maintain human relationships. For example, when a man presents an engagement ring to a woman, it is a gift and not a payment. So, too, Christmas presents to children are gifts (unless they have been corrupted by being described as payment for "being good"). So, too, are gifts to teachers, priests, and friends (schools, churches, and communities).

Money and other gifts are always exchanged as a way of creating and maintaining marriage, parenthood, and all social relations. This exchange of gifts is not "payment for services rendered," but it is the ritualized form for bringing into existence person-to-person relations which are themselves the condition for the furtherance of human life. To assert that there should be no money exchange involved in activities maintaining personal relations (I-Thou), but only in relations between persons and things (I-It), is an absurdity. To say that the I-Thou relations should be "free" and that only I-It relations should involve the exchange of money is to be confused about the basis of social life. There simply is no problem with the exchange of money to establish or maintain any surrogate or marital relation *as long as that money is exchanged as a gift, or as a compensation for lost time, rather than as a payment for services.*

In Vitro Fertilization

The reason why the ethics of *in vitro* fertilization have not been discussed heretofore in my essay (nor in most of the essays in this volume) is because it did not arise as a question during the Baby M trial. That is, the court did not regard the "form of conception" as a matter for its consideration. The issues it focussed on were (a) the status of the contract between Mrs. Whitehead and the Sterns, and (b) the question of the custody on the basis of what was best for the child. Therefore, the opponents of the practice of *in vitro* fertilization have not been able to express, in this volume, their own deepest concerns to the extent they confined themselves to commenting on the issues discussed in the case itself. It is only fair, therefore, that the topic of *in vitro* fertilization be introduced now.

I am not a Roman Catholic ethicist (but a Calvinist). I do not speak for the Catholic Church. But I want, at this point, to try and explain (and defend) one of the basic concerns behind the Catholic opposition to *in vitro* fertilization and to contraception. To begin, ask yourself this question: "When I *intend* to conceive (or not to conceive) a child, what am I doing?"

When I intend to conceive a child (as, in *in vitro* fertilization), am I thinking that I can create a child in the same way that I think I can create a chair? That is, is my idea of procreation similar to my idea of manufacturing? Do I *intend* to make something when I *intend* to get (someone) pregnant? *If so, then I am thinking of children as products of my own activity.* Once I have started thinking of them in this way, how can I regard them as free subjects possessing dignity and rights?

I am perfectly aware that many (if not most) people think of children as their property. I watch people spank and batter their children as if they were pieces of furniture (or worse). I watch parents describe children as if they "belonged" to them. (We are just beginning to realize that adult wives are not property—so habituated are we to this mode of thinking.) It takes a certain intellectual and spiritual development to be able to think of children as persons and not as property belonging to oneself (or one's race!). The beginning of that development is to know oneself as a person, as a spiritual being. One cannot treat others as persons if one does not know and treat oneself as a person, that is, if one does not know from self-knowledge what a person is. Therefore, the beginning of understanding the problem of *in vitro* fertilization is not a rational argument, but a personal enlightenment.

If one knows oneself to be a spiritual being, possessing freedom, and knows one's child is also such a being, then it follows that one will not imagine that we can produce or manufacture children. That is, we know that children are not the products of our will nor do they exist because we intend them to exist. What this means, in short, is that one realizes that *sex does not create babies*. Sex may be the condition of their conception. *But babies are conceived because of something else.* In traditional language, that "something else" is God.

The Catholic arguments against *in vitro* fertilization and contraception are attempts to maintain the condition for right thinking about the origin of human life. That is, the Church states that both conception and the avoidance of conception are not proper intentions, or goals, of the sexual act. In sex, we should neither intend to conceive nor intend not to conceive ("the contraceptive mentality"). According to the Catholic view, we should not *intend* conception because it is not we who create life, but someone else. We should allow our sexual activity to remain "open" to the divine intention. God alone has the right to intend human creation and we respect this right by not intending it ourselves.

This Catholic argument does articulate a reason why we should regard all human life as "sacred" and as "possessing inalienable rights." Human life exists, it says, because God intended it and created it. Human life does not exist because *we* intended and created it. Human life is not manufactured by us; it is given to us—as a gift to be cared for. Therefore, the Catholic viewpoint presents an adequate (perhaps the only adequate) foundation for a society in which the rights and dignity of all persons are inalienably secured.

An Alternative Approach?

Could there be, however, an account which would understand the dignity and rights of every child to derive from something antecedent to society without resorting to a theory of "nature" such as is employed by the Catholic Church? Must we, in accepting the idea behind the Catholic theory, also accept the Catholic repudiation of contraception and *in vitro* fertilization? Could we provide an alternative account of the "sanctity of human life" which would be compatible with certain of the advances in technology that we today take for granted? I think it is possible.

Let us begin by asking "When, and in what way, do human beings become persons with inalienable rights?" If such personhood and rights are bestowed by society, then why may society not take them away? If the right to exist and to be treated as a person is not yours from the beginning of your existence, then why could these rights not be taken away? From these considerations, it seems that we must acknowledge persons possess these rights and their dignity from the very beginning; rights are not later bestowed upon persons by society. That rights are acknowledged to be possessed by human beings from the beginning of their existence evidences that society regards these rights as deriving from some power which is "higher" than itself.

Where did Baby M get those rights which Judge Sorkow acknowledged when he said that the custody issue had to be settled in *her* best interest (rather than the interest of either her genetic mother or her genetic father)? The court's acknowedgement that Baby M possessed full human dignity involves it in a rhetoric which is in total contradiction to the rhetoric used to describe her *in vitro* conception. According to the rhetoric of the court, Baby M is a person with a dignity equal to any other person. According to the rhetoric of the medical science which produced and implanted her, Baby M is a product of human purpose and engineering. How and when did the transition from one description to the other description take place?

It is, of course, a commonplace to say that different specializations utilize different vocabularies and that there is no necessary contradiction involved in employing different descriptions of the same event. Yet it seems to me that, in this case, the differing descriptions do tend to be antagonistic, impeding our ability to think clearly about the problem. If these descriptions really are contradictory, then it may be that we have only two choices: the Catholic Church or Auschwitz. Is there any third way?

Let us return to consider the activity of human procreation to see if we can describe it in a way which preserves what we seek (the dignity of the *conceptus*) without needing to employ the middle levels of argument from "nature" which are used by the Church. Can we describe procreation so that it is associated with the creation of persons rather than with the production of products? I have argued that the Catholic argument is successful in its description of procreation because it denies that the creation of persons (i.e. conception) should be defined as a *goal* of the sexual act. That act, says the Church, should not aim at conception nor at the avoidance of conception, but should remain "open" to its possibility. The conception, if it takes place, occurs not because we intend it, but because God intends and effects it. By this argument, *the Catholic Church presents sexual intercourse not as the cause of conception, but as its condition.* The cause of conception is something other than the sexual act. The cause of the conception is God, who creates the child "as a living soul" (or "person").

I believe that the Catholic Church is correct in affirming that each child is created immediately by God. What this means is that each person exists as a "child of God," as a spiritual being immediately related to God. Each person has a spiritual value and destiny. This is not only the view of the Catholic Church, but of all Christian Churches—indeed, of all religions.

The Catholic Church defends its affirmation that God creates each person by arguing that the act of intercourse is not a *cause* of procreation, but a *condition.* In conjunction with this condition, God sometimes acts to create new life. But we should ask exactly what it is about sexual intercourse which qualifies it to be the appropriate condition for God's creation of human life.

The reason, I suggest, that sexual intercourse is the appropriate condition for God's creation of life is that sexual intercourse is the most expressive and focussed form of *human love.* It is not the act of sexual intercourse which constitutes the condition which God blesses with the conception of new life; rather it is the love between two persons, uniting them through the act of intercourse, which God blesses with new life. It is in conjunction with the expression of love between a man and a woman that God bestows the gift of a child. God "crowns" love with this blessing.

I understand that many people find this way of looking at the matter to be absurd. For them, conception results from sex—and love has nothing whatsoever to do with it. But the argument must be made that, among persons, it is love which gives to sex its meaning and its character. This is so much the case that sexual intercourse is described as "making love." More importantly, this quality of sex as "love" is not found in "nature," but is only found among persons who are spiritual beings.

In Behalf of *In Vitro* Fertilization

The love between persons which can be expressed in the act of sexual intercourse is not tied to that act alone. Rather, this love can be the character of a total relation, affecting all aspects of the interaction and life of the couple. If it is there, in the total relation, then it is also there in the sex act. If it is not there, in the total relation, then it cannot be there in the sexual act. If love is not there, the act of intercourse does not express love. It is just sex.

My reason for arguing that love is the characteristic which makes sexual intercourse the appropriate condition for God's creation of new life is to suggest an alternative to the Catholic description of sexual intercourse *per se* as the natural condition for God's creation of a child. The Catholic view asserts that sexual intercourse should remain "open" to conception. What this means is that conception should not be the intended *goal* of intercourse. This implies that the purpose of intercourse should be something other than conception, *something intrinsic to the act itself.* I agree with this position. I agree that sexual intercourse should not intend conception or to block conception. Sexual intercourse should intend to be what it intrinsically is: an act of love. This love can be a *condition* in relation to which God can create new life.

My argument is that, between persons, the *purpose* of sexual intercourse should be to unite them in love. This love is an end in itself; it does not intend a product beyond itself. Therefore, as the form of human union, love also establishes the condition to which God can respond with the gift of a child. In this way, a child's conception is separated from the order of human productive activity. In this way, the child's dignity and rights will not be conceived to be *derived* from us, and, therefore, removable by us.

But if the qualifying condition for conception is human activity which creates and expresses love, then this love need not be identified only with the act of sexual intercourse. Rather, this love may also be expressed through a variety of other acts—such as *in vitro* fertilization. I fail to see why the actions of thinking, planning, attending appointments, arranging agreements, and going through the lengthy medical procedures which conclude with *in vitro* fertilization are any less "love" than the act of sexual intercourse. If love is the qualifying condition of conception, then *in vitro fertilization may fulfill this condition as well as the act of sexual intercourse.* Therefore, *in vitro* fertilization is a means no less legitimate as a condition of conception than the more "natural" (which only means more "usual") sexual intercourse. In fact, since the proper condition of conception is *moral action* (not material action), it may be that *in vitro* fertilization allows us to ascertain the presence of the "love" as the qualifying condition better than intercourse itself.

One might object that *in vitro* fertilization does not seem to be a *condition* of conception, but actually aims to be a manufacturing process producing babies. If this is so, then we must reject it as morally wrong—for this would bring us back into the world of the "baby factory." *But this is neither a necessary nor a correct interpretation.* In fact, *in vitro* fertilization (no less than sexual intercourse) can seek the establishment of a condition in relation to which God may act to create children. There is no reason at all why God may not be conceived to act in relation to such scientific activity if God may also be conceived to act in relation to nature and to natural activity. *In vitro* fertilization may, therefore, be regarded as a "religious service."

What Professor Deegan earlier proposed in relation to the money exchange in the surrogate relation (namely, that it be ritualized as a "gift") anticipated what I am here proposing in relation to *in vitro* fertilization. The activities of medical technology are susceptible to both religious and to materialistic interpretations. There is no reason why we need to regard science as being in conflict with religion; and it is difficult for me not to interpret medical techniques which assist persons to fulfill the conditions for conception, the creation of children, as anything other than in a religious way. When persons who love act to establish conditions in relation to which God may grant them a child, that is almost a form of *prayer*.

Science Assists Nature

In my own tradition, the Calvinist, "nature" is not regarded as an inviolable normative good. Rather, the Calvinist tradition stresses that nature, no less than persons, is "fallen." This means that there is a mixture of good and evil in both persons and nature. In persons we find compassion and hatred, hope and despair, openness and pride, knowledge and ignorance. In nature we find both health and disease, vitality and impotence, wholeness and defect, birth and death. The religious problem is to overcome the destructive elements in life. In Calvinism, the power of God is understood to work towards the transformation of evil so that the intended full goodness of creation can be restored. Therefore, in Calvinism, science is the means by which God works to restore goodness to nature, to establish "the kingdom of God on Earth." On this view, the work of science is linked with the religious task.

Of course, science may be taken over and used by anti-human forces so that it becomes not a blessing, but a curse. The use of scientific power apart from, and against, the spiritual purpose of all life makes science demonic. But the misappropriation of science from its true purpose, from its partnership with religion, does not change the fact that science can be a form of God's sovereignty for the sake of redeeming nature so that it will serve the human good. *In vitro* fertilization is a way that science can help us to fulfill God's command to "be fruitful and multiply."

My own reflections on the strength and value of Catholic moral teaching about conception make me hesitate before pointing out the Calvinist disagreement with the Catholic understanding of nature and of science. Yet, it is precisely where the issues of "the normativeness of nature" and "the scope and responsibility of science and technology" are joined that the Catholic and the Calvinist traditions are not in agreement. The Catholic tradition regards nature as rational, integral, and good; therefore, the Catholic tradition is very wary of technological intervention. The Calvinist tradition regards nature as contradictory, broken, and evil in many ways; the Calvinist tradition is, therefore, committed to technological intervention aiming at the improvement of the conditions of life.

Two views of nature, involving different conceptions of the task of science and technology, are embedded in our history. The Catholic view, affirming the sanctity of nature, continues the Greek tradition. The Calvinist view, denying any holiness in nature and stressing, over against nature, the will and purpose of a transcendent God, derives from the Hebrew tradition. Yet both traditions, Catholic and Calvinist, are in full agreement that God is the direct creator of all human life and that all persons possess the full dignity and rights of "God's children." This is the basic affirmation that these—and all!—religious traditions defend against the materialistic accounts of the procreation of children as "products."

An Ecological Evaluation of Surrogacy
A Wrong Idea for Our Time

MARCUS P. FORD AND SANDRA B. LUBARSKY

At the basis of the ecological sciences is a complex notion about the relationship between an individual organism and its environment. This complex notion includes the belief that an organism is inextricably linked to its environment, not by a single thread but by a web of connections, for an organism's environment is everything that affects it. And the reverse is also true, an organism affects its environment, not in any single way, but always in a myriad of ways simultaneously. If, for example, one thinks about a tree in a forest, from an ecological perspective one cannot think about it independently of its environment--the condition of the soil, the other forms of vegetation, the animals that inhabit the forest, the air quality, and on and on. Nor can one think about the forest, the soil, the wildlife, or the air apart from the individual tree. For the tree is affected by everything in its environment, and in turn affects everything in its environment.

The appropriateness of the ecological perspective, we contend, is not limited to what is often referred to as the natural sciences. Cultural phenomena must also be viewed as webs of causal relations. Ideas, inventions, institutions, works of art, and other cultural manifestations, arise out of a matrix of earlier ideas, inventions, institutions and works of art, and their influence, however limited, is never limited to a single incident or individual.

When thinking about the phenomenon of surrogate motherhood, one needs to think ecologically.* One needs to look at the current conditions that constitute the present environment and one needs to consider what effects surrogate motherhood might realistically be expected to have on the various social and biological realities that constitute our environment.

The widest environment of all surrogate cases is the global one. All of us live on the same planet and what one person does affects all others. By the time this article appears in print, the human population of the planet will be five billion. Less than seventy years ago, the population was under two billion. Fifteen years from now, barring a nuclear war, the population will be six billion. A century from now it will be ten billion, or twice what it is now. It is true that the vast majority of this increase will occur outside of the United States of America and that most of the immediate effects of overpopulation will be felt first in these other, mostly third world countries. However, it is also true that because of the high standard of living that we Americans enjoy, any increase in the population of the United States has a greater impact on the global environment than does the same increase in population in a "less developed" (or at least a less consumptive) country.

When intellectually abstracted from the global situation, surrogacy might be viewed as a novel institution that will help some and hurt no one. In fact, all increases in population have some effect on all of us, and some of these effects are hurtful. Moreover, it should be noted that, at least as it is currently being practiced, surrogate mothering is a very expensive practice. When all is said and done -- when the doctors and the lawyers and the surrogate mother are all paid -- the cost can exceed forty thousand dollars. Were our planet underpopulated and were there unlimited resources, and if there were no harmful social consequences of surrogate mothering, then there would be nothing wrong with promoting such an institution. But this is not the case.

---

* The term "surrogate motherhood" is unfortunate since it reduces the meaning of motherhood to its biological aspects and disregards its social aspects. As will become clear in what follows, we hold that the biological notion of family is an insufficient notion and hence the term, "surrogate motherhood," does not sit well with us.

Although the global situation is in fact very concrete, its complexity is such that most of us tend to disregard it. Most of the time most of us make our decisions as if the rest of the world simply did not exist. It does, and it needs to figure into how we think about things, including surrogate motherhood.

Still the global environment, although the most inclusive, is not the only environment that needs to be considered. The narrower, or most immediate, environment of surrogate motherhood is family life in our own nation. We can make a meaningful move from the planetary unit to smaller social units precisely because of the network which holds human life together with all other life. To repeat our basic assumption, our lives are not lived apart from the lives of others (both human and non-human others). Families are webs of relationships within larger webs of relationships, within larger webs, and so on. The ecological perspective is not different from the "personal" perspective or the "sociological" perspective. The principles that apply in the one, apply in the other.

Because we began with the concern for global ecology does not mean that our concern for individuals, in this case the Sterns and the Whiteheads, is lessened. The significance of our lives, and in particular our family lives, is not diminished when seen from within a global ecology, but heightened. From an ecological perspective, we are not first individuals who subsequently come together to form families, rather we are the product of families. By "family" we means a web of relationships that both binds human beings together and provides the substance for an individual's individuality. From the ecological perspective, the family life is absolutely fundamental.

In what follows, we shall look briefly at three concepts of the family: 1) the biological notion of family; 2) the legal notion of family; and 3) the "organic" notion of family. We shall argue that a family is not, at its roots, a biological unit or legal entity. Rather, a human family is a web of relations, best described organically. It is within the biological notion of family that surrogacy seems to be a reasonable option; it is within the organic notion of family that surrogacy is undesirable.*

An important argument raised against surrogacy is that it undermines the family. But what concept of family life is being assumed here? In the particular case of Baby "M" a great deal of attention is focused on the biological notion of family. The court opinion includes the belief that, "The desire to reproduce blood lines to connect future generations through one's genes continues to exert a powerful and pervasive influence" (p. 12) and that, "This desire to propagate the species is fundamental" (p. 73). More specifically, the court opinion includes the fact that Mr. Stern lost most of his family in the Nazi Holocaust and that he is now the sole survivor on both his mother's and his father's sides. This fact deserves attention only if one assumes, as both the biological and the traditional notions of family do, the overwhelming importance of bloodlines. But is it really the case that the desire to produce bloodlines, to be genetically linked to the future, exerts an irresistable and pervasive influence over all individuals? And if it is true, should this desire be encouraged at all costs, even at a time of overpopulation? Furthermore, shall there be no distinction made between "the desire to produce blood lines...*through one's genes*" and the "desire to propagate the species?" While the desire to

---

* The term "traditional family," currently popular with fundamentalist Christians and political conservatives, is most closely linked with what we are calling the biological and the legal concepts of family. The so-called "traditional family" is usually, though not always, biologically connected and virtually without exception in accordance with the legal statutes. But the notion of the "traditional family" includes more than biological connectedness and legality. In addition to these things, the "traditional family" is one in which the father is head of the household, where the mother has primary responsibility for cooking, washing, childrearing, community work, etc. etc., and the children are, above all else, respectful of their parents. Much of what we say about the biological and the legal notions of family will apply to the traditional notion of family, since the traditional notion of family includes the biological and the legal notions.

propagate the species may be fundamental, the desire to do so with one's own genes may not be. The biological account of family fuses the two urges together and thus it seems to be the case that if the one desire is restricted—the desire to reproduce one's particular genetic information—the other desire is undercut—the desire for species survival. But in fact, this is not necessarily the case, and in our world, the reverse might even hold true: survival of the human species demands reproductive restraint. Are those people who practice such restraint, who willingly choose not to have children, biological anomalies? If the biological notion of family is to serve us well as an explanation of our behavior, it must answer these (and other) questions.

If it is assumed that the basic notion of family is the biological notion (an assumption that we are challenging), surrogate mothering would appear to be one of the logical options open to infertile couples (for single males, or couples who for medical or non-medical reasons decide not to gestate their own offspring). Of course, if one assumes that the basic notion of the family is the biological notion, the surrogate mother is not merely the "birth mother" or the "natural mother," she is quite simply the mother in exactly the same sense that the genetic father is the father. But the biological notion of the family, can be used every bit as forcefully to argue against surrogate motherhood as it can be used to argue for it. For surrogate motherhood contributes to the building of some families—biological families—only at the expense of diminishing other families. In this particular case, the Sterns' gain is quite literally the Whiteheads' loss.

A further difficulty with the biological notion of family (one that has been noted above in regard to the desire to reproduce one's genes) is that biology, the science of life, is itself a cultural artifact. There is no escaping cultural bias in the interpretation of observed or hypothesized facts. Anyone familiar with Aristotle's biology and Bacon's knows all too well that biology can be and has been sexist biology.* Although contemporary biological theory is much less

---

* An excellent overview of the history of science in regard to its cultural and sexist bias is Carolyn Merchant's book, *The Death of Nature: Women, Ecology, and the Scientific Revolution* (Harper & Row, Publishers, 1980.

blatantly sexist than earlier biologies, one could argue that the earlier biologies are the ones that have had the greatest impact upon our cultural common sense. One example of how sexist biology still plays a dominant role in our society is that almost without exception it is the male bloodline or "seed" that is seen to be essential, and the maleness of this is compounded by the fact that the bloodline is usually thought to be guaranteed only if the offspring is a male. In patriarchal societies, the woman's role in procreation is less than the man's: the seed rules the egg. In a culture in which the norms are male-determined, the intense desire to propagate the species has been become the intense desire to continue male bloodlines. We are no longer talking simply about biological replication. On a planet that is dangerously populated with the human species, in a world in which there are unwanted, unparented children, how can the practice of surrogacy be justified? It can be justified only by a cultural imperative, arising from within a partriarchal culture and given precedence over biological demands.

Another manifestation of sexist biology is that of the objectification of woman -- the bias toward seeing women as mere means, and not also as ends. The verb "to conceive" has traditionally functioned in two ways, determined along the lines of gender: men think, women reproduce. The association of women with physical being, with matter, and with nature but also with passivity, with lack of internality -- all of this has resulted in the objectifying of women. Most recently, the birthing woman has experienced this loss of selfhood most intensely within the primarily male institution of the hospital. She has been looked upon by health practitioners as a means to an end and the quality of her "birthing experience" has been keenly neglected. She is an object to be sanitized, monitored, and numbed. In surrogacy, a woman is more thoroughly objectified. Mary Beth Whitehead is, in the surrogacy arrangement, solely a means to an end. She is not the wife of the father nor shall she be able to mother the child. As things now stand, she does not acquire a new role, equal to or better than those she forfeited under the surrogate contract. Until (and if) a new and cogent role can be formulated for the surrogate, she is a *persona non grata* in the surrogacy affair. She who is undergoing one of the most critical human experiences, that of carrying and delivering a child, is reduced to an "it."

If there are good reasons to reject the biological notion of family as fundamental, what about the legal notion? The legal notion of family is, for the most part, a formalization of the biological notion of the family, but not entirely. It is also a nest of abstractions concerning how individuals ought to behave in regard to each other. From the legal perspective, a family is a set of legal and financial responsiblities and obligations. Parents are legally responsible for their children's welfare and for their children's actions; spouses are responsible for each other's debts; and so on. The legal notion of the family, in our opinion, is the reification of the organic notion. Relationships, the very stuff of life, are extracted from the web of experience and thus become abstractions. In the legal formulation, a contract is the primary reality. How can it be otherwise? The legal system is an attempt to generalize, to systematize, to categorize, to depersonalize. It is a very abstract endeavor. When the law describes the family, it produces a one-dimensional, mechanical picture. Until very recently it has legitimized the objectification of wives and children as property of husbands and fathers. It may talk in detail about obligations of economic support, but cannot address obligations of psychological or emotional support. It speaks in terms of rights and obligations and not in terms of love. The abstractness of the legal system is evidenced in its inability to be inclusive of a larger whole. Families consist of blood relations or adopted relations. That is all. If you lived for 20 years with your best friend, you are still not family. Someone who took you in and raised as if you were their own child is not, legally, family. A close friend of the family's someone you've always known as "Aunt" or "Uncle," in the eyes of the law, does not exist as such. For all its complexity of language, the law does not, and cannot, capture the complexity of reality. And it is this intrinsic inability to mirror the concrete interconnectedness of things that renders the legal notion of the family a useful abstraction, but often a dangerous one.

Having rejected both the biological and the legal notions of family as fundamental, we must now consider what we are calling the organic notion of family. The organic notion of family operates on the metaphysical assumption that the relationship between individuals is based on something more basic than genes and that is "feeling." We need not be genetically linked in order to feel ourselves to be deeply a part of another person. The technical term used by the philosopher Alfred North Whitehead is "prehension." He writes, "Actual entities [the fundamental units of the world] involve each other by reason of their prehensions of each other." In the process of prehension, the other loses her/his externality and becomes literally a part of our selves. Such feeling is the basis of all intimacy.

Certainly not all feeling is the same level of intensity. There is a web of existence because there are feelings or prehensions, but some events are more strongly connected to each other than other events. (And they need not be spatially connected.) The members of a particular society, for example, need not share a genetic inheritance, but belong to the same group because they are, in some important ways, alike. They have "a liking" for each other, arising from a shared inheritance. In less modern societies it was often the case the people referred to those who lived in the same society as family. The Mohawk Indians, for example, considered everyone who lived within their longhouses to be family, although that included other than blood relations. Although it is less the case now, until recently many Jews considered their family to be the world Jewish community and were intensely committed to people they knew not at all

With our American culture, it is most often the case that one's strongest feelings are directed toward members of the same biological unit. Children are told that "blood is thicker than water," that "no matter what," your sister/brother is still your sister/brother. And yet many of us grow up and find that we have more in common with our friends than with our siblings and that we feel closer to our friends. What sense does it make to continue to see the one as family and not the other? Our point here is that there is a degree of randomness operative within a culture that emphasizes the bond of blood over all else. There is a sense in which we are "thrown" into our particular family units; it is assumed that those with whom we share a certain genetic lineage will necessarily constitute our significant others. Without doubt this arrangement gives an essential degree of order to our society. The notion of the organic family is not a complete rejection of the notion of the biological family. Rather, it pushes beyond the limited degree of order maintained by the notion of the biological family and in doing so lessens the degree of randomness at work in our culture. The notion of the organic family reflects the belief that our lives are connected with all other lives and although the sense of connectedness may be strongest between biological relations, it is a mistake to so limit this connectedness. There are many ways in which unities can be formed, and there are higher levels of ordered complexity that can arise. Truely we live in a global community; let our notions of intimacy reflect this more clearly. If we do not, we move more quickly toward self-destruction. Perhaps we will be charged here with sentimentality in contending for the "brotherhood of man" (sic). But there is metaphysical justification and ecological and political motivation for doing so. The nuclear age demands the higher type of order, of relevance, of responsiveness, of coordination that the organic notion of family can provide. Our call, then, is for the realization, on the most familiar level, of our personal involvement in the human family.

The organic notion of family is that of a group of people tied together, not necessarily by blood or by law, but by commitment. A family is a group of people committed to each other, a group of people who love each other, who are willing to share each other's triumphs and failures, who are willing to sacrifice for each other, and so much more. Members of a family, in the organic sense of the term, may be biologically related. Indeed, the experience of giving birth can and ought to be a powerful experience that binds the parents together with each other and with their children. But a family, in what we take to be the most basic sense of the term, can exist independently of biological relatedness and independently of birthing experiences. A family, in short, is a group of people who are held together by a web of relationships. Or, to emphasize another aspect of the organic notion of family, a family is a group of people who contribute to the very being of the individuals in the family in a significant and usually productive manner.

Surrogate motherhood (or, more accurately, prearranged adoption of a genetically-related child) undercuts what we understand to be the most fundamental sense of family, the organic meaning, by giving undue credence to the biological and the legal notions of family.

In lieu of surrogacy we advocate adoption. There is, unfortunately, no shortage of young people who desperately need parents. At the present time adoption is more difficult than it ought to be. Partially this is the fault of those who wish to adopt: many Americans limit their desire for children to a desire for newborn, Caucasian, unquestionably heathly children. And partially this is the fault of adoption agencies who maintain outmoded notions of who would make good parents. (One such outmoded notion is the policy that the adoptive couple be under 40 years of age.) There are further difficulties that arise when international adoption is attempted. These are serious problems that need to be resolved for all of our sakes. Surrogate motherhood arrangements only circumvent these problems and thus indirectly exacerbate them, while simultaneously creating additonal and original social problems. In this world whose population is rocketing toward ten billion human beings, surrogacy needlessly worsens the situation. There is, to our shame, no shortage of children who need loving parents and there are people who want to be parents but are biologically unable to do so. Ways must be found to bring these new families into being.

In some other world, or in our world some time in the distant future, there may come a time when surrogacy will have to be looked to as the best option. If, for example, there were a nuclear holocaust that resulted in the death of billions of people and the sexual sterilization of hundreds of millions of "survivors," under these conditions surrogate mothering would make a good deal of sense (though we would object to the surrogate mother receiving payment for her services). But thankfully these are not the conditions that prevail in human ecology today, and hopefully they never will be. Surrogacy, from our ecological perspective, is not in itself wrong; it is only wrong for this world in these times.

SYMPOSIUM SERIES